about bi?ethics

CARING FOR PEOPLE WHO ARE SICK OR DYING

Nicholas Tonti-Filippini

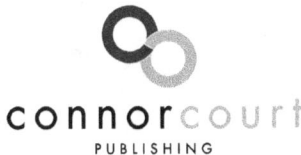

About Bioethics - Volume 2: Caring for People who are Sick or Dying

Published in 2012 by Connor Court Publishing Pty Ltd.

Copyright © Nicholas Tonti-Filippini, 2012

All rights reserved. No part of this book may be reproduced or transmitted in any form or by any means, electronic or mechanical, including photocopying, recording or by any information storage and retrieval system, without prior permission in writing from the publisher.

Connor Court Publishing Pty Ltd.
PO Box 1
Ballan VIC 3342
sales@connorcourt.com
www.connorcourt.com

ISBN: 9781921421785 (pbk.)

Front cover design: Ian James

Scripture quotations, unless otherwise noted, are from the Revised Standard Version of the Bible.

Excerpts of Vatican documents are from the English translation found on the Vatican webpage: www.vatican.va.

Printed and designed in Australia.

Also in this series:

About Bioethics
Volume 1
Philosophical and Theological Approaches

by Nicholas Tonti-Filippini

Contents

Preface	1
1. Caring Relationships	**11**
1.1 A Relationship: Not an Industry, Not Just a Service	11
1.2 The Patient's Right to Say "No"	29
1.3 Truth-Telling in Health Care	38
1.4 Professional Conscience	47
1.5 Justice and the Allocation of Scarce Health Resources	63
2. Care ... Until the End	**71**
2.1 Care of the Dying and Proportionate Means	71
2.2 Not for Resuscitation Orders	76
2.3 Tube Feeding	79
2.4 Refusal of Food and Water	84
2.5 Euthanasia	95
2.6 Physician-Assisted Suicide	102
2.7 The Fragility of Living a Burdensome Life	107
3. Representation and Disability	**121**
3.1 Best Interests Decisions vs. Substituted Judgement	121
3.2 Options for Planning Future Care	138
3.3 Accepting Death and Dying	139
3.4 Desirability of Future Care Planning	140
3.5 How is a Representative Appointed?	141
3.6 What to Record?	142
3.7 Why Guide the Representative?	143
3.8 More about the Problem of Advanced Directives	144
4. Ethics and Mental Illness	**149**
4.1 What is Mental Illness?	149
4.2 Classifying Mental Illness	151
4.3 The Significance of a Diagnosis	152
4.4 Truth telling and Diagnosis of Mental Illness	154

	4.5 Ranking Psychiatric Treatments by their Capacity to Alter Personality	155
	4.6 The Social Uses of Psychiatry	156
	4.7 Families and Confidentiality	157
5.	**Being a Patient**	**159**
	5.1 Love, Empathy and Suffering	159
	5.2 Living with Disability and Chronic Illness	173
Bibliography		**201**
Index		**207**

Preface

What I have attempted in this volume is to consider the various issues that are debated in Bioethics, about the nature of the relationship between health professionals and those who depend on them in sickness and dying, and to contrast that formal discussion with my own narrative of faith and love in response to the personal experience of illness, and encounters with human frailty and human goodness in my role as an ethicist. I hope that readers are not surprised by the juxtapositioning of formal analysis of issues with personal anecdotes.

We live in a secular culture that embraces some post-enlightenment liberal doctrines as a background for post-modernism, and the dominance of the individual narrative. Against that secular culture, the idea of a universal ethic, such as is promoted by natural law theory, and most recently discussed in those terms by the International Theological Commission, appears as a modern anathema.[1] In pursuing the notion of a human person and a thick notion of the human good, natural law is simply not on the same page, so to speak, with contemporary culture. There are some, such as the communitarians, Charles Taylor for instance, and others, who have, to some extent, bridged the gap between secularist individualism, on the one hand, and a "master narrative" of positive freedom, goodness and virtue, on the other, but in the main there is not much of a secular dialogue that is open to natural law ideas, despite the robust philosophical defences of it by contemporary thinkers such as Alasdair MacIntyre, John Finnis, Germain Grisez, Joseph Boyle, Robert George, Russell Hittinger, John Haldane, Steven Long, and Martin Rhonheimer. There was a brief time, post World War Two, when the notion of a master

---

1 I believe I owe this line of thinking to many conversations with Tracey Rowland and her criticisms of the International Theological Commission *The Search for a Universal Ethic* discussed in volume one.

narrative in the form of a law above civil law[2] found expression in the *Nuremberg Trials* and the origins of the modern human rights movement. In his 1963 encyclical *Pacem in Terris,* Pope John XXIII appealed to four basic concepts: truth, justice, charity and liberty that engaged the international willingness to consider natural law. The encyclical was an effort to dialogue on the basis of a consensus about natural law as the law above civil law.

However the window did not stay open long. By 1973, Maurice Cardinal Roy advised Pope Paul VI that this notion of nature had been very much questioned or rejected for its essentialism.[3] The contemporary human rights movement has replaced a thick theory of the human good with overriding respect for autonomy, subjectivism and the consequent loss of the sense of the sacred, as anything other than a religious term. The personal narrative has supplanted the master narrative.

In that context, I am offering a narrative of my own faith and love as a personal response to the issues, while seeking to give an account of the issues that upholds the dignity of the human person as someone who is always to be loved. There is a tendency for contemporary codes of ethics to be minimalist – a set of standards below which no-one should venture. Instead, my view is that ethics should explore what is the ideal in human relating in a given circumstance. I take heart from the National Health and Medical Research Council which under the chairing of Dr Kerry Breen and then Prof Colin Thomson had adopted an ideal relationship approach to the *National Statement on the Ethical Conduct of Human Research* (2007), replacing the previous minimalism.

It is not a question of just being a passably good clinician or researcher, but rather, what are the ideals of the therapeutic relationship to which health professionals might aspire, and how best might

---

[2] This was formalised when in 1950 the United Nations International Law Commission adopted the Nuremberg Principles. The basic premise of the principles is that no person, no matter what their office, stands above international law. http://www.wagingpeace.org/menu/issues/international-law/start/un-nuremberg-principles.htm.

[3] Cf. Russell Hittinger "Evidence Lost and Found: Concluding Scientific Postscript" *Nova et Vetera* Summer 2011, Vol 9, No. 3, pp. 825-842.

we, as patients, cope with illness, suffering and death? I offer a personal answer to those questions.

In the preface to volume one, I offered some autobiographical comments and choose not to repeat them here, although they apply especially to this volume, because much of this volume reflects my own journey with illness, and my encounters with others on that journey. Enough is also said on personal matters elsewhere in this volume.

Volume one discussed *Philosophical and Theological Approaches to Bioethics*. That also frees me of the burden in this volume of explaining a theoretical approach to Bioethics. Essentially, the experience of serving on government committees and conducting public consultation has affected my view about how to develop Bioethics policy, and the way in which, through discussion and seeking consensus, we can transcend individual perspectives and construct guidelines that reflect ideal relationships between clinicians and patients, or between participants in research, as researchers or the researched. There are commonalities in the human experience that allow us to develop an ideal of the ways in which we flourish, and the importance of protecting the opportunities for human flourishing for each individual.

The origins of the contemporary human rights movement did just that in deriving its catalogue of equal and inalienable human rights from the idea of inherent human dignity.[4] The latter concept is more likely to provoke embarrassment or resistance in contemporary culture. Dignity as it was used in the 1960's context is a very rich concept given the content of the rights it generates, and is inclusive of respect for the person, the worth of the person and their freedom, values and culture. To support it is not to endorse cultural relativism: far from it, the presumption is that there are truths of human experience which are reflected across the different cultures, and that by working with

---

4 See the preambles to the *International Covenants on Civil and Political Rights:* http://www2.ohchr.org/english/law/ccpr.htm and on *Economic, Social and Cultural Rights:* http://www2.ohchr.org/english/law/cescr.htm.

others we can seek to transcend cultural influences through the use of reason without, however, every denying the influence of culture and language upon us. The human rights instruments do not represent a particular culture, rather they represent human beings and what they have and need in common.

As Alasdair MacIntyre[5] suggests, we can seek to arrive at an understanding of the human good, and of moral acts, that is robust to reasoned analysis and not dependent on any particular viewpoint. I have suggested in volume one, that a faith perspective should offer its conclusions to that process. The particular idea of love as gift of self, that is taught and exemplified by Christ Jesus, is a robust notion in itself, and believers need have no fear that it might not withstand rational analysis.

Christians believe in a God of love who, in creating us, set us free in an intelligible universe. Christianity thus nurtured science and reason, and the scientific project of seeking to understand the universe as an intelligible order, in which every effect has a cause. We value science because, in helping us to better understand nature, science helps us better understand ourselves and the Creator. The Catholic Church did not reject Darwin's evolutionary theory, holding instead that evolution of the species could be consistent with belief in divine creation of the universe.[6]

The Church recognises a partnership between faith and reason, but that they operate in different spheres. The norms of investigation that apply to the visible, do not apply to the invisible (Colossians 1:16). Scripture was written according to the knowledge of science of the day. It is not a scientific text. It is, however, an account of the history of the relationship between God and humanity.[7] I discuss this issue at length in the volume *Ethics, Creation and the Environment*. Science on the other hand cannot explain why we exist and provide

---

5 MacIntyre, Alasdair *The Tasks of Philosophy: Selected Essays*, Vol. 1, CUP 2006, esp. Ch 7.

6 See for instance: Pope Pius XII, *Humani generis*, 1950, n. 36.

7 Ratzinger, Joseph *In the Beginning... A Catholic Understanding of the Story of Creation and the Fall* (English Translation) Our Sunday Visitor: Huntington, Indiana 1990.

purpose and meaning for illness, sickness and death. Faith proposes to do so.

In many ways, this is a very personal volume, setting out an account of my own views of illness, disability, suffering and dying, as a philosopher, but one who is influenced by my own faith, but open to hearing what others contribute. I do not think, for a moment, that I have, or the Catholic faith has, all the answers to every ethical question, despite my respect for the scholarship in faith and in reason, which the Church represents.

So much of what is encountered in Bioethics is new, and requires fresh solutions that, though respecting age old truths and norms of behaviour, still require development. In that regard I admire Cardinal Newman's concept of doctrinal development[8] and the freedom it gives to scholarship within faith. Newman recognised that there had been and continues to be doctrinal development, but as a building on doctrine not a refutation of doctrine. He writes in *An Essay on the Development of Christian Doctrine in 1845,*

> To discriminate healthy developments of an idea from its state of corruption and decay, as follows:—There is no corruption if it retains one and the same type, the same principles, the same organization; if its beginnings anticipate its subsequent phases, and its later phenomena protect and subserve its earlier; if it has a power of assimilation and revival, and a vigorous action from first to last.[9]

In other words genuine doctrinal development does not supplant, but is rooted in the old. That leaves us with the scholarly task of comparing new ideas with the old, as growth from, rather than supplanting the old. I am always fascinated by what I see as doctrinal development in which an older form of expression is replaced by

---

[8] Newman, John Henry, *An Essay on the Development of Christian Doctrine,* Longman's Green and Co. London, New York and Calcutta 1909.

[9] Newman, John Henry, *Op. Cit.* Chapter 5, Para. 4 http://www.newmanreader.org/works/development/chapter5.html#section4.

a deeper understanding, rendering the older expression no longer representative of the consistent truth.

For instance, we find in the 1930 encyclical *Casti Connubii* n. 59 reference to the quieting of concupiscence as a purpose of marriage. The concept has not since been repeated in papal teaching, because it seems to conflict with a contemporary understanding of what marital love means, in the Scriptural analogies to divine love, and in distinguishing between love and mere use. We seem to have moved to a deeper understanding of long held concepts, in which love, and mere use as an object, are inconsistent.

There has been a development of doctrine, with respect to marriage, that better reflects the Scriptural truth, and which has the power of assimilation and revival as we are seeing in the Theology of the Body of recent times. There is therefore a dynamic process occurring, of doctrinal development.

As I outlined in volume one, if we do not listen to others, of faith or of none, and are not open to their contribution, then we have no right to expect to be heard. A truly democratic society welcomes the contributions to discussion of public policy and law reform from all parts of society. No-one, and no group, should be excluded. There are politenesses and norms of public discussion that should be followed. However, in the common effort to ensure that whatever consensus develops is as well informed as it can be, we should be completely open to the different views and ready to accept or reject them on the basis of reasoned analysis of what is proposed, and not on the basis of who proposes it.

The tragedy of contemporary secular society is the closed-mindedness of those who, in the name of secularism, see fit to declare that those of faith have no contribution to make to public discussion. However, I discussed religion in a secular society at length in volume one.

Much of what is in this volume developed as lectures to graduate students. Though I have modified and adapted the material for a broader audience, I have maintained the norms of academic scholarship, while also adding my own personal narrative.

In this volume, in the first set of essays, I have addressed the nature of the relationship between patient and health professional, arguing that health care should not be seen as an industry, or just as a service. The need in health care ethics is to give an account of the nature of a relationship between the patient, who is dependent on care, lacks the knowledge, expertise and experience of the health professional, and may have some disability through the illness, and is thus exposed to an unequal situation of vulnerability, and the health professionals who engage with him. The importance of ethics is in offering guidance to the participants in that relationship, so as to preserve the equal dignity of both parties.

The second set of essays addresses the care of the dying, and includes analysis of the issues involved in not for resuscitation (NFR) orders, artificially delivered food and nutrition, overly burdensome or futile treatment, the different forms of euthanasia, and the debate over making some forms of euthanasia lawful.

In the early 1980s, NFR orders were often informal, sometimes an asterisk on a whiteboard, or on the nursing chart, sufficed. The decisions were seldom well documented, often for fear of legal consequences. At times they took the form of a go slow order – make the call but do not hurry. It was a major task, as an ethicist, to encourage discussion and to be part of the conclusion that a clear and well documented decision, following consultation, was much less of a risk for everyone, than what had been the practice. Documentation meant having a clear protocol, and I was very privileged to be part of the St Vincent's Hospital committee process to develop a set of guidelines for NFR orders, including discussion with the patient or the patient representative, the indications for a resuscitation order and the documentation requirements. To my knowledge, that first set of guidelines for NFR in the 1980s soon operated in at least 18 hospitals.

Recently, I experienced being approached myself with the question as to whether, if I suffered a cardiac or respiratory arrest, I wanted to be resuscitated. I would not have been approached in the unfortunate manner I was, and with such inappropriate timing, had the original St Vincent's guidelines been operative where I was. I was, at the time, acutely ill in intensive care, and not in a position to deal adequately with the question, and the timing only served to dishearten, in what was a battle to survive against an acute respiratory infection – not the advanced degenerative illness that normally gives rise to the question about whether resuscitation would succeed, and whether it would be overly burdensome. I discuss this matter further in section 5.2.

In the third set of essays, the issue of representation in the circumstances of disability is addressed. There is currently a battle between idealistic individualism, on the one hand, and the communitarian needs and situation of people who are dependent on the assistance of others. Currently, Victorian law has adopted a best interests principle that includes the values, wishes and culture of the person who is represented. The individualist challenge to that proposes what is called "substituted judgement", which greatly reduces the possibilities for having the representation reviewed in the best interests of the represented person, and consequently gives much greater authority to the person who is the representative.

In that section, there is also discussion of future healthcare planning and advanced directives or living wills. There are great problems when the law upholds and enforces advanced directives issued with a relative lack of knowledge of the eventual circumstances, and thus not representative of informed consent. The better course for people to take is to appoint someone to make decisions, when, and if, they become unable, and to ensure that they have discussions with that person or persons about their wishes and values to be applied, depending on the circumstances. That leaves that person free to represent the person's wishes and values in the actual circumstances, but to do so in conjunction with discussion with the treating personnel, with relevant information and in recognition of any ethical difficulties that might present. An advanced directive can make uninformed, inappropriate or unethical demands because so much is unforeseeable.

The fourth set of essays discusses mental illness and some specific problems that arise. Mental illness is in a different category from other areas of medical ethics, precisely because, often enough, the illness leads the person to have wishes and values that are not reasoned and not in their best interests. So the values and wishes of the person, that would normally be so important in the making of decisions, may need to be overridden in order to treat, in the person's best interests, but against their immediate wishes. The ethical justification for such measures is the belief that the illness is impeding the person's ability to function, and the goal of treatment is to restore their function by treating the impediment. Also, the decisions still should be in accord with the patient's belief and values – when not so impeded by illness. Such decisions need to be reviewed, and special care needs to be taken to protect involuntary patients.

The fifth set of essays is much more personal, giving an account of the problem of evil – why suffering exists and its relationship to empathy and love from my own perspective, and drawing on experiences of illness and the relationships that came to be or were affected by my illnesses.

Because there is much that is experiential in this volume, I wish to acknowledge and dedicate this volume to my wife, Mary, who has stood with me in all of my illnesses and often suffered far more than I have in her medical knowledge of what was happening. Often she endured the waiting, while I was blissfully anaesthetised or otherwise unaware. That experience of empathy through difficult times has greatly deepened our love. Mary has also been a constant support and source of medical advice in the writing of these volumes, as well as being a critic and editor. I also acknowledge and dedicate this volume to our four children, Claire, Lucianne, Justin and John, who have lived with me and my illnesses, and years of dialysis, throughout their childhoods, coped with the wash-back of my public roles, and been a major part of forming who I am, through our struggle to be adequate parents. Parenthood is an experiment with unconsenting human participants in dependent relationships, that would never be approved by a Human Research Ethics Committee. I can only apologise for the many mistakes that I made and trust in their understanding of my love for them. I fear that the older children suffered much more from my mistakes than the younger, but the former also had the advantage of our relative youth and energy.

I also wish to acknowledge the John Paul II Institute for Marriage and Family for the sheer joy and privilege of teaching graduate students who are so keen and so dedicated, and my colleagues who are so much involved in shaping and informing my ideas, Bishop Peter Elliott, Professor Tracey Rowland, Dr Adam Cooper, Dr Gerard O'Shea, Dr Colin Patterson (who came from being my student to being a valued colleague), Colonel Toby Hunter, our Registrar, and Anthony Coyte, our Publicity and Promotions Officer. There are many others who have contributed, but I have provided a more comprehensive set of acknowledgements in volume one.

Subsequent volumes have been written, and are currently forthcoming, on organ and tissue donation, ethics and human sexuality, motherhood and technology and finally a collection of issues such as capital punishment, just war theory, torture and cooperation in evil. I have also just completed a set of eleven graduate lectures on *Ethics, Creation and the Environment* to be edited for inclusion in the set as volume seven. I may be able to match JK Rowling and her Harry Potter, for the numbers of volumes, even if not her popularity.

Professor Nicholas Tonti-Filippini
BA (Hons) MA (Monash) PhD (Melb)
FHERDSA KCSG
Associate Dean and Head of Bioethics
John Paul II Institute for Marriage and Family

1. Caring Relationships

1.1 A Relationship: Not an Industry, Not Just a Service

1.1.1 Introduction

Cars, washing machines and other devices are made and serviced. Industries are formed for the purpose. People, on the other hand, are not industrial products, they are not objects. Their care is a relationship between people, those who have needs and are dependent, on the one hand, and those with professional competence, knowledge, skills and commitment, on the other. It is not an equal relationship, so preserving respect for equal and inherent dignity requires effort.

The late Archbishop Eric D'Arcy wrote:

> To picture healthcare as an industry is to entertain a false model. Since it concerns the lives and the pain of human beings, and the vocation of those who care for them, the distortion can be cruel … [I]t would be a tragic day for Australia's sick and helpless. Some aspects of health care resemble those of an industry: for instance their care is wages, salaries, holidays, hours, rosters, maternity leave, superannuation, and similar matters... In the case of health care, however, one sees at work a strong tendency to slide from … treating it as if it were an industry to the fiction that it really is so... A patient in a hospital or a resident in a nursing home is not the object of an industrial process, no matter how advanced or refined this may be. Every human being is unique. No human being is simply the clone of another. The development of every person is an entirely individual history. On the other hand, the epoch-making Industrial Revolution of the 18th and 19th centuries had, at the very heart of its success, the ability to turn out the same thing over and over again. Every product is identical with every other product of a given industrial process: when the process hiccups, you simply

discard or throw away the defective ones. This is the very opposite of healthcare.[1]

Healthcare is about caring for people and that relationship between health clinician and patient develops its own character depending on the characters involved.

In contemporary hospitals they have discovered that they can save money by removing gender distinctions so that men and women find themselves sharing rooms and bathrooms, their beds side by side, and no privacy from the many questions asked, and discussions had, about the state of one's various bodily functions or the lack of them. The utilitarian thinking that ignores the significance and sensitivity of gender is most unfortunate. However, it did mean that as a patient I have often observed the interactions between patients and health care personnel not because I wanted to do so, but because it was unavoidable. Even if a screen is drawn, the interactions are public knowledge. It often fascinated me how the interactions differed.

I recall a situation recently in which four of us in the room had respiratory infections and renal disease – they grouped by disease and not gender.

Lung infection may be viral, bacterial or fungal in origin. One prays that it is not the latter as the treatment is the most difficult. In any case, there is an urgency to treat as a lung infection may be a life risk. However, identifying the particular bug involved can take several days of culturing in the laboratory before something recognisable grows. Further, whatever does grow in the laboratory may simply be coincidental and not the source of the illness. If antibiotics or anti-viral treatments have already been started before sputum samples are gathered, then the bug causing the problem may be prevented from being cultured in the laboratory. Basically, it is trial and error, applying antibiotics or antivirals that work for the more common bugs and then moving on to other agents, if those do not

---

[1] Eric D'Arcy "Healthcare is not an industry" *Bioethics Outlook*, Vol 22, No 3, September 2011.

produce signs of improvement, until something works (or nature heals or death intervenes!). In the meantime, clinical examination, and the various forms of scanning track the progress of the disease. If lung function is significantly compromised then it can be a battle to maintain survivable levels of the blood gases. That was the battle that I found myself in for a brief two days in intensive care. Afterwards, while recovering, I shared a room with four others, as I mentioned.

At that time, there was a regular track of the various teams – renal, respiratory and infectious diseases, each with a very similar set of questions to ask and treatment decisions to be made, though we were each at different stages of disease process. Despite the similarities of process for diagnosis and treatment, it struck me how very different the interactions were. Each of us had very different types of interaction and different ways of assimilating information. There were also significant differences of approach by the various teams and team members.

One patient took control over the relationships, examining the tablets that the nurse put out for her, wanting to know what each was (they often look different from different manufacturers), and checking to ensure that it was appropriately prescribed. She would question the team, rather than have them question her, and openly compare any advice offered to what she had already been told. She did so humbly, rather than challenging, implying that it was her difficulty in understanding, rather than inconsistencies in the advice given. She took a very active role in what happened and her positive attitude to illness, participation in decisions, and general cheerfulness were inspirational, despite the setbacks that she experienced and the frustration of an illness not responding to treatment. Despite the embarrassment of sharing a room with someone not of the same gender, I greatly appreciated her presence, and the benefit of being a witness to her strength as well as discussing shared literary interests. At the same time I regretted that she had to suffer my male presence, and invasion into her privacy, and the noise of my coughing day and night.

Another patient with renal disease and a lung infection, an elderly man, had so much more to bear as he also had multiple sclerosis (MS) which was advanced so that every task, even turning over, required assistance, and speech had become difficult. He said little about his treatment decisions and asked few if any questions, but was an avid contributor to discussion of his diet despite the effort that speech required, and a keen follower of sport which he discussed at length with his visitors. His calmness and acceptance, in the face of such disability and dependence, made me feel small.

The third was a former soldier and appeared the sickest of us at that time. He was at the early stage in which they were trying treatments without much amelioration of the infection, but causing him quite severe side effects. He too took little part in treatment decisions except to ask for help with nausea and vomiting, which appeared to be what was causing him the most distress, despite the severe nature of his lung infection and his general state of weakness. I could identify with that as earlier I had myself experienced a very uncomfortable symptom that was my major concern, but the least of concerns for the treating team who were understandably focussed on oxygen saturations levels and survival. He was going through a dreadful time battling both the disease and the severe side effects of the treatment, but uncomplaining, unquestioning and compliant.

Four characters each with different relationships to the teams requiring different responses, despite similarity of illnesses. One of the thoughts that occurred to me later was how far removed much of this was from informed consent. I may have missed it, in the circumstances, but I do not recall any of the team warning me of the list of common side effects of the various treatments that were tried. Generally, the first information of a side effect was in fact experiencing it and having the nurse or physician nod sagely when I reported it and indicate that yes that is one of the side effects. Decisions were made about which agents to try and in what sequence and obviously they were doing some balancing of the relative toxic nature of the treatments and their effectiveness, but as the patient struggling for breath I had little or no involvement in those decisions, apart from being asked whether particular agents had been used in the past and reactions to them on other occasions. Mary was more involved than I was, but I do not recall the kind of sequence that the informed consent legal dogma would require. The reality was the need to treat, and as a patient I did not need to know the complexity of their decisions other than that they would keep trying different agents until something worked. It may be better not to know the likely side effects. Placebo effects are real. If one may be nauseated, vomit, or develop a painful rash, joint pain or a migraine, it does not help to be awaiting it: far better to deal with the effects only when, and if, they make their unwelcome presence felt.

On the other side of the therapeutic relationship, the members of the teams were very different. There would often be a senior consultant, a registrar and a resident, making a daily round together, and at other times, the individual members returning on their own or in company. When as a team, the senior consultant would usually conduct the conversation with the patient, occasionally holding a discussion with the juniors. Some consultants would adopt an overseeing role, leaving the more junior doctor to conduct the engagement with the patient. There were very different approaches to the patient. Some would begin with reporting to the patient some salient details of what was in the nursing and medical notes, test results and the like, and the implications to be read into them, rather like an interview with the headmaster on one's unsatisfactory progress. At some stage, they would then ask the patient for an opinion on what had been decided.

Others would begin the consultation by asking the patient what was happening, and what was expected, and then refer those answers to the notes for clarification. Some would begin with a physical examination, asking questions of the patient as they went, and explaining what they had found in the examination and how that related to the information on record including the tests results. Again, different characters forming quite different relationships, and giving the patient different roles and opportunity to participate. Most would make their own individual clinical examination, and exchange notes on what they had heard with their stethoscopes. In some approaches, one felt as though one were the recipient of a decision made by others. In other approaches, one felt as though one were a partner in the decisions. In others, one felt as though one was being expertly assisted and advised to make one's own decision from the options presented. In that order, the three approaches roughly coincided with the theoretical ideas of *paternalism* and *authority*, *fiduciary* relationships, and *contractual* understandings of the doctor-patient relationship. Thankfully, none coincided with what I would call a *free-market*, take it or leave it, approach. (See discussion of the differences in section 1.3 below). All three approaches had a clear idea of seeking the best treatment, in the circumstances, and unambiguous treatment goals and concern to achieve improvement. There were also niceties about issues of authority between teams. Strictly, I was admitted as a renal patient and the renal team was primarily responsible for my care, even though different matters fell under the different areas of expertise of the respiratory, infectious diseases and cardiac teams respectively.

The conversations about discharge from hospital are interesting – who initiates the conversation, and what factors are to be taken into account? Often there are policies, such as no discharge within 24 hours of a fever. It seems that it is a black mark against the team if a patient is subsequently readmitted. Casemix funding has guidelines about what are considered *inliers* (discharged within the prescribed timeframe) and *outliers* (discharged, early or late, outside the prescribed timeframe for a diagnosis) and the funding formula applied penalises the hospital for outliers.[2]

---

[2] I have discussed the effects of casemix funding elsewhere. See for instance: Tonti-Filippini, Nicholas "Blame Casemix: Not Just the Budget Cuts" *Quadrant* June 1995; Tonti-Filippini, Nicholas "Casemix is bad for patients" *Social Action*, No. 147, February 1995.

I try to get out of hospital as soon as it is safe to do so for several reasons: while I am in hospital Mary is under strain, tracking back and forth from home and spending hours waiting on uncomfortable chairs, then frantically busy when she is at home catching up on the things that need doing; second, the reasonable fear of exposure to hospital-based infection in an immune-compromised state; and third, I find hospital beds with their plastic covered foam mattresses uncomfortable, the rooms too noisy to permit much sleep, and hospital wards very claustrophobic. Because of the latter, I battle an underlying sense of panic much of the time. I always find myself longing for the space of home within reach of the outside, a comfortable bed, and a quiet and a decent sleep. Also I suffer from episodes of pleuro-pericarditis which can be quite painful. The management has been good with a sophisticated range of treatments prescribed to control it and reduce the symptoms. However, in hospital, despite cooperation and understanding from the nurses, the formal process of making the treatments available as prescribed can be time consuming and require some forward planning with the pharmacy. The waiting can be difficult.

Despite all the differences in the relationships formed in healthcare between patients and health professionals, the relationships in healthcare have a singular focus – on health. The niceties of the relationships may cover other matters, but the goals of investigation and intervention relate to health. That professional commitment is both significant and welcome but may be endangered within post modernity as I discuss below.

1.1.2 Defining Health as the Focus of the Relationship

Health has proven to be quite a difficult concept to define. We may have a rough idea that it means soundness of body and being free from illness or ailment. We also apply it to narrower concepts such as mental health or reproductive health. More broadly we may refer to spiritual health, but that is not always the focus of professional healthcare. There are also broader notions of health with respect to how one sees the human person, and how one answers questions about the nature and existence of mind, body and soul.

One aspect of health is its relativity. A person with a chronic illness or a disability may have a very different idea of what constitutes health for them, from someone who lacks chronic illness and disability. A chronically ill person may say that he or she is well, or healthy, as a concept that pays no regard to the chronic illness, and refers only to what may be changeable, such as whether he or she has an infection at that time. Similarly a frail aged person may have a multiplicity of illnesses and disabilities, but consider themselves well, relative to their normal level of dysfunction and discomfort.

One seemingly contradictory concept is healthy dying,[3] or living with dying,[4] which may be used by those engaged in palliative care. They may have a particular notion of what is healthy within the dying process.

The World Health Organisation defines "health" as "a state of complete physical, mental and social well being and not merely the absence of disease or infirmity."[5]

There are problems with the definition: notably that a state of complete physical, mental, and social wellbeing corresponds much more closely to happiness than to health. Health and happiness are distinct experiences and their relationship is neither fixed nor constant. Having a serious disease is likely to make you less happy, but not having a serious disease does not amount to happiness. Common existential problems – involving emotions, passions, personal values, and questions on the meaning of life – can make your days less than happy or even frankly uncomfortable, but they are not reducible to health problems.[6]

---

3 Neuberger, Julia "A healthy view of dying" *BMJ*. 2003 July 26; 327(7408): 207–208.
4 Berzoff, Joan, Silverman, Phyllis, *Living with Dying* Columbia University Press: New York 2004.
5 World Health Organisation, *Basic documents*. 39th ed. Geneva: WHO, 1992.
6 Saracci, Rodolfo "The world health organisation needs to reconsider its definition of health", *BMJ* 1997; pp. 314:1409 (10 May).

On the other hand, the experience of illness can have many complex aspects that at times may seem inseparable from the meaning of ill-health. First, there is the impact on function, effectively causing disability or reduced ability. Second, a factor that causes suffering and frustration is its unpredictability, which causes uncertainty and insecurity and a sense, and the reality, of loss of control and mistrust in one's own body.

Linked to serious illness may be a reasonable fear of dying, fear of greater disability or fear of greater pain. I have written in the final chapters about pain and suffering, and about the distinction between chronic and acute pain. The irony is that the pain experience may be the same in any given situation, but, because of the risk of drug tolerance, the medical care of chronic pain may be quite different.

With illness and disability may go dependence, and people may react very differently to the associated loss or change of role in their relationships within the family and wider society. Illness may mean loss of employment, financial insecurity and hardship. Loss of status can be, for some, the hardest factor with which to cope. Further, insecurity and pain are both disabling in themselves. Someone who is used to being in control of his or her life, and perhaps the lives of others, may find it very difficult to have to accept not being able to plan ahead. It can be quite difficult to switch to living a day, or even an hour at a time, with illness not having a definite finish date, and symptoms fluctuating unpredictably. The response may be depression and not being able to take advantage of the opportunities that come between disabling symptoms. Coping well with illness and disability means accepting what befalls, but also welcoming those moments of greater opportunity when the vagaries of the disease process grant a reprieve.

In cultures that experience machismo, men may find illness challenging to their self image and their mode of relating. That too can be depressing. In some cultures, matriarchs or patriarchs may assume control of the life of someone who is ill, and the latter may become passive, even childlike, in the cultural role of being sick. Italian men may react that way, and in some Islamic families health care decisions may be taken by the senior male in the family. I observed some fascinating difficulties with doctors at St Vincent's seeking to apply the concept of informed consent in circumstances in which, within a family, culturally the decision-making role fell to someone other than the patient. The legal niceties were met by seeking consent from both, though confidentiality issues were complex.

I also did some work in relation to drafting ethical guidelines for research involving Australian Aboriginal people, or Torres Strait Islander people, and have discussed some of the difficulties with palliative care in those communities. One difference, and there are many, is that there is a much stronger notion of community which has a bearing on consent issues, and the concept of reciprocity may play a role. There may also be issues of spirit and integrity that an outsider may not comprehend.

1.1.3 Dying and Sharing a Good Death

Another difference in communities of Australian aborigines is that attitudes to death may involve apportioning blame for the death in the belief that someone must be responsible. I found it curious that there was a similar notion recorded in the literature about ancient Greece. If that is the cultural belief, then the normal palliative care process, of beginning the process of accepting the dying process, and seeking to live as fully with it, rather than futilely pursuing curative treatment, may drive family members away, at that time when relationships may be so much more important.

Knowing that one is likely to die, in the not so distant future, can be rich in meaning as people adjust to the changed circumstance and often find so much greater depth and meaning in their relationships. As the individual relinquishes hold on this life and its priorities, and turns to thinking of the next life, or life in which they are not, those present with them may be privileged to experience that change within them. There is often great tenderness that develops because the relationships may lose their competitiveness, and many people may discover aspects of each other and their friendship that were not evident because previously, the factors of living life, and life aspirations, blocked them.

For Christians, the theological virtues of faith, hope and love have a special place at this time, giving us confidence in our welcome by an all-loving God, a confidence nurtured by the sacraments, which are signs of God's presence in our lives, and sources of divine grace. I have several times experienced what we call "anointing of the sick" and the "Eucharist" together. They are both sacraments of reconciliation, of finding peace with God. For me they brought also peace within myself, in accepting what God wanted for me, and the knowledge that I was secure in his love.

The idea of taking control of that dying process and seeking to engineer death at a time of one's own choosing, i.e., euthanasia or assisted suicide, are discussed later.

1.1.4 Illness, Death and Relationships

What I think is crucial in understanding illness and death is that the human person exists in relationship with other persons, with the world, and with himself, and, for a believer, with God. Illness affects those relationships and death profoundly alters them.

Contemporary culture seeks to privilege the idea of autonomy, and so the loss of autonomy that can be the result of illness and the dying process may be an anathema. Some would rather be dead than lack autonomy.

I understand, but do not share the view. I dread losing rational function through pain and suffering and other aspects of illness, and I have had many such experiences. I have even on occasion expressed a preference for death, rather than what I was enduring. Recently when battling lung infection, an intensive care nurse advised that it was either manage to get oxygen levels up by my own machine-assisted breathing effort, something I found difficult and exhausting, or they would need to opt for anaesthesia and full intubation. At the time I felt that the latter would be most welcome, even though as I understood it, the complications of anaesthesia may have risked death in those circumstances. But the thought was only passing because I was not alone. At every step of that difficult time, Mary was beside me and it was of her presence that I was most conscious. I knew that I should continue to battle because of her and the children, confident in their love and the sense that we have so much more life to share, especially the desire to share together with Mary in their joy when in the future they may make some major decisions, such as to love someone else. (I used to pray that I would live long enough to see the last child, John, complete his schooling, feeling that by then my primary responsibility as a parent would have been completed. Now that that has been reached, I have discovered further targets!)

There were some repeated demands made by a senior intensive care nurse, at one point, that Mary as a family member should leave during the crisis, despite her being a medical doctor, and I felt enormously relieved when she took advantage of the crowding of the room and doorway (they had made a call for emergency assistance) to stay where she was. I desperately did not want to be alone and without her tangible loving presence. Love means many things but empathy, and its great significance, is humanly irreplaceable, as I discuss in the final section.

1.1.5 Imago Dei

Beyond those relationships that I mentioned, which will keep me striving to stay alive until the means used become either futile, in that they do not do so, or overly burdensome in that the treatments are just too awful, there is the puzzle of my relationship as a believer to my Creator and Saviour.

I may be criticised by fellow Christians at this point for my failure to acknowledge God's love, the other theological virtues, and divine grace with respect to His carrying me through these times. Divine grace is a mystery to us. We do not know what role the Creator may be playing in our lives. We may pray for great, life-changing miracles, but I suspect that in being surrounded by the miracle of human love, I have been given miracles enough, despite moments when I failed to appreciate it or was driven by the fear or the desperation of pain and illness.

The International Theological Commission referred to the belief that the body is an intrinsic part of the human person, and thus participates in his being created in the image of God. This is a central dogma of the Christian faith. "The Christian doctrine of creation utterly excludes a metaphysical or cosmic dualism since it teaches that everything in the universe, spiritual and material, was created by God and thus stems from the perfect Good. Within the framework of the doctrine of the incarnation, the body also appears as an intrinsic part of the person".[7]

When I am suffering a significant episode of illness, I have found that I may not feel as close to God as I should or as conscious of God's love as would seem appropriate for a believer. I am however always conscious that Mary is God's image and likeness. It is a curious aspect of Christian marriage, that we bring each other closer to God, through seeking to love as God loves.

As a Christian I accept death, believing that my immortal soul shall cease to animate the matter of my body, and life shall cease to be until I am resurrected. For non-believers that may seem far-fetched but that is the core of my belief. We do not believe in bodies without souls because the soul is needed to maintain the unity and integrity, the integration of the body. (See volume three on organ donation). The Commission writes:

> ...the DNA of the chromosomes contains the information necessary for matter to be organized according to what is typical of a certain species or individual. Analogically, the substantial form [the soul] provides to prime matter the formation it needs to be organized in a particular way.[8]

---

7 International Theological Commission, Op. Cit. *Communion and Stewardship: Human Persons Created in the Image of God*, n. 28.
8 Op. Cit. n. 30.

> Human bodiliness participates in the *imago Dei*. If the soul, created in God's image, forms matter to constitute the human body, then the human person as a whole is the bearer of the divine image in a spiritual as well as a bodily dimension. This conclusion is strengthened when the christological implications of the image of God are taken fully into account.[9]

The Second Vatican Council affirmed, "In reality it is only in the mystery of the Word made flesh that the mystery of man truly becomes clear… Christ fully reveals man to himself and brings to light his most high calling."[10] Pope John Paul II expressed a related idea, "As an incarnate spirit, that is a soul which expresses itself in a body and a body informed by an immortal spirit, man is called to love in his unified totality. Love includes the human body, and the body is made a sharer in spiritual love"[11]

I do not relish for one moment the thought of losing the precious relationships to Mary, my children and others. But I also trust in God's love and immortality with Him. It is a leap of faith, but not unreasonable to believe that there is a loving God who loves every one of us. Nevertheless, it is not something that I expect to prove to a non-believer, nor even expect her to accept. I do not believe that reason can yield all the conclusions of faith, but I do believe that what I believe as a matter of faith is not contrary to reason. Accepting that something requires faith is not the same thing as saying that faith is contradicted by reason. Something can be consistent with reason, just not proven by reason.

What I do hope, though, is that others who do not share this belief, may see not just the happiness in the theological virtues of faith, hope and love, but also the calm acceptance that it brings of the prospect of death, despite not wishing or wanting to suffer in the process, nor wishing to lose the loving relationships of this life. The things that are

---

9 Ibid., n. 1.
10 *Gaudium et Spes*, n. 22.
11 *Familiaris Consortio*, n. 11.

ultimately important for a believer are not trapped in this existence. We can genuinely let go, albeit humanly reluctantly, especially our love for those so precious to us.

We can dialogue also about what letting go might mean for someone who does not share our faith, and hence does not necessarily share the theological virtues. Faith or otherwise, there is a need to accept illness, suffering, disability and death, and we benefit enormously from relinquishing the less important things of ordinary life, and sharing the joy and release in so doing with our loved ones, assisting them to be part of our journey of life, and helping them to gain perspective about what really is important in life, as we finally seek to live as fully as possible with the dying process. In our dying we continue to serve others, no matter how helpless we become in the process.

1.1.6 Healthcare Principles

That we *can* do something does not mean that we *ought*. There are questions that face everyone about: How far may science go? How far may science go in an attempt to remake mankind? What is essential to the individual human identity of each of us and not to be altered? How do we ensure responsible stewardship of our universe, and our planet, particularly, but also of ourselves within it? A right to dispose of something extends only to objects with a merely instrumental value, but not to objects which are good in themselves, i.e., ends in themselves. The human person is herself such a good.

The focus of healthcare, as I argued earlier, is on each person and in caring for them, and relationships are formed. What does it mean to respect the person? Is her body an object, open to manipulation, or an icon, something not to be altered?

In Catholic tradition are some principles that have brought real comfort as people negotiate decisions about the care of their bodies and their mental health. I offer them as defensible in preserving the focus of health care on caring for the human person, including his body.

There was a time when the Church developed a manualist tradition of simple principles that suited confessors who might not have been competent, or well enough trained to undertake the reasoning needed to resolve difficult moral dilemmas, or to assist someone to know that what they did may be entirely consistent with love of God and neighbour despite the appearance otherwise.

The first of them is the principle of stewardship, which the writers of the Middle Ages tended to base on the belief that life comes from God, and humans are "stewards", responsible for the care of the body. Fine for believers, but can more be said about this for those who do not share that belief? I am of the view that we can. We do think of managing the environment sustainably. We think of this in terms of protecting it for future generations. That is to say we exercise stewardship of these resources for those who are to come. That is not just about sustainability, it is also about preserving pristine wildernesses and about preventing loss of habitat that would result in loss of species. There also is a sense in which species, wildernesses and other parts of our environment are not just valuable because someone in the future may value them. It is hard not to see one of the wonders of nature without a sense of awe and preciousness. Within that environment are human beings, part of the same natural world, something of a pinnacle of evolutionary processes, especially with such human capacities by which we reason, doubt, wonder, affirm and ultimately love. Do we need God to tell us that we are precious or can we see that for ourselves? When a young person unknown to us dies in an avoidable motor accident, or a soldier from a roadside bomb, can we not all share in that sense of great loss?

Finally, is a world that requires stewardship of human life a worse world than one that sees life as expendable if it loses its utility? Which culture would one prefer to belong to or live as a person with chronic illness or disability? This is particularly pertinent to the euthanasia debate, and what I later discuss as the fragility of living a burdensome life with respect to euthanasia policy.

A second principle relates to the first. It is the principle of the inviolability of human life and states that innocent life may never purposefully be taken in actions such as abortion, suicide, or euthanasia. This is a debate we have had over and over again without resolution. I discuss it extensively in a volume on Motherhood and Technology so will not go into great detail here.

Most supporters of abortion do not say that the foetus is worthless, or that abortion is a good thing. Rather, the acceptance of abortion for many is an acceptance that it is a matter that the woman should be able to choose, and the law should protect her choice. In a book[12] I co-edited with John Fleming, we published some research, by independent consultants, into Australian attitudes. One of the conclusions was that the vast majority of Australians favoured making the woman's choosing lawful, but at the same time indicated their *moral* disagreement with the reasons why most abortions are performed. In other words morality and the law are separate in their minds. It struck me that there is a great deal of common ground on the moral questions, even if views are polarised on the legal issue. There was also majority acceptance of measures such as opportunities for independent information and counselling.

A third principle is the principle of totality that allows us to regard each part of the body as existing for the good of the whole, and therefore limbs, for example, may be amputated if it is necessary to protect the rest of the body. The meaning of this principle is that the human person develops, cares for, and preserves all his physical and mental functions in such a way that (1) lower functions are never sacrificed except for the better functioning of the total person, and even then with an effort to compensate for what is being sacrificed; and (2) the fundamental faculties which essentially belong to being human are never sacrificed, except when necessary to save life.[13]

---

12 John Fleming and Nicholas Tonti-Filippini (ed.), *Common Ground? Seeking an Australian Consensus on Abortion and Sex Education*, St Paul Publications: Sydney, 2007.

13 ITC, Op. Cit., n 83.

The principle of totality may be defended as an application of double effect reasoning and similar cautions apply:

- There must be a question of an intervention in the part of the body that is either affected or is the direct cause of the life-threatening situation;
- There can be no other alternatives for preserving life;
- There is a proportionate chance of success in comparison with side effects; and
- The patient must give assent to the intervention.

1.1.7 Goals of Healthcare

What makes healthcare a profession is that it is a commitment to serve the health needs of the patient. It is important that health care professionals remain professional, committed to the good of body and mind of their patients, otherwise they would just be technicians. They must have clear goals that define what the profession is and does. Therapeutic interventions serve to restore the physical, mental and spiritual functions, placing the person at the centre, and fully respecting human teleology, the reason why a person exists.

Some particular goals of health care include:

- To promote health and prevent disease
- To deepen our understanding of the causes of disease and to develop new forms of treatment
- To save life, cure illness or slow the progress of disease
- To relieve suffering and discomfort
- To care for people when they are sick, disabled, frail or elderly
- To assist a person in his or her transition from this life in hope of resurrection, while also caring for those who grieve for that person.

Having clear goals defines what the health professions are and their committing to them is essential to the community being able to trust the health professions. It is remarkable that in Australia, unlike in the United States, our medical institutions do not expect graduates to make a commitment, such as the Hippocratic Oath. It is tragic that since the early part of the last century, there has in fact been nothing to indicate that they are part of a guild or tradition that is honoured for its values. Instead, some faculties have encouraged students to formulate their own declaration, but there is an absence of any formality or any commitment to a common mission or professional values.

In this volume, I discuss the impact of the health professions serving definite purposes of healthcare, and the relationships formed between health professionals and their patients with respect to health. What is the right thing to do in any given circumstance is both expressive and formative of that relationship. It is important that we do not see codes of ethics as mere sets of rules, but in fact guidance as to how best to conduct that relationship. Codes of ethics should reflect an ideal in human relating, and not just be a lowest common denominator of minimalist standards.

1.2 The Patient's Right to Say "No"

1.2.1 Consent and Refusal

In Australia, the relationship between a health professional and a patient assumes that the patient's participation is voluntary. This is often expressed as the obligation to obtain informed consent. As I will explain in this and the following section, the latter is complex: it is a duty to inform and a duty to offer reasonable care options for the patient's acceptance. The exercise of those duties is often not straightforward and in the practical circumstances of healthcare, frequently treatment needs to commence before the difficult process of achieving a complete understanding by the patient can be achieved. I prefer to express the patient's role in this process as a right to be informed and a right to refuse treatment because that seems to more accurately describe what happens in practice, despite the recent adoption of the notion of informed consent as apparent ethical dogma.

The right to refuse treatment is recognized in law in all Australian jurisdictions, with some limitations. There are exceptions made for emergency treatment when there is too little time to explain the implications of a refusal to the patient (or the relative, or other representative, of a person who is too affected by illness or trauma to be able to speak for him- or herself). There are also exceptions made in some jurisdictions where the patient displays suicidal ideation, and the medical intervention is considered part of a response using reasonable force to prevent suicide, where there is a reasonable belief that the person intends suicide.[14] The Victorian *Crimes Act* 1958 contains the provision:

> **463B. Prevention of suicide**
>
> Every person is justified in using such force as may reasonably be necessary to prevent the commission of suicide or of any act which he believes on reasonable grounds would, if committed, amount to suicide.

In the Act, a related provision prevents adding and abetting suicide:

> 6B. Survivor of suicide pact who kills deceased party is guilty of manslaughter
>
> 1. Where upon the trial of a person for the murder of another person the jury are satisfied that the accused caused or was a party to causing the death of that other person by a wilful act or omission but are satisfied on the balance of probabilities that the act was done or the omission made in pursuance of a suicide pact then the jury shall, notwithstanding that the circumstances were such that but for the provisions of this section they might have returned a verdict of murder, return a verdict of manslaughter in lieu thereof.

---

14 Most Australian jurisdictions have an exception to the *Crimes Act,* such as the above, to permit the prevention of someone with suicidal ideation from doing so. Those who attempt suicide and are brought to the emergency room are treated to attempt to save their lives.

1A. Despite section 5, a person convicted of manslaughter under subsection (1) is only liable to level 5 imprisonment (10 years maximum).

The New South Wales *Crimes Act* 1900 contains the following provisions:

Prevention of suicide

574B Prevention of suicide

It shall be lawful for a person to use such force as may reasonably be necessary to prevent the suicide of another person or any act which the person believes on reasonable grounds would, if committed, result in that suicide.

31C Aiding etc suicide

1. A person who aids or abets the suicide or attempted suicide of another person shall be liable to imprisonment for 10 years.
2. Where:
   a. a person incites or counsels another person to commit suicide, and
   b. that other person commits, or attempts to commit, suicide as a consequence of that incitement or counsel, the first mentioned person shall be liable to imprisonment for 5 years.

Attempting suicide is no longer a criminal offence, but aiding and abetting it remains an offence, and there is no need for consent to act to prevent suicide.

Normally, however, consent is legally required for a medical intervention, even if the treatment is in the patient's best interests, except for the two circumstances mentioned above. In practice, consent is often implicit rather than a formal event. Doctor (nurse or other health professional) and patient engage in an interaction in which treatment is discussed and, in the absence of any indication to the contrary by the patient, consent is assumed. Even where there is a formal consent process such as signing a consent form to anaesthesia and surgery, it is open to the patient to indicate to the contrary at any stage. In practice therefore, the concept being applied is an on-going right to refuse rather than a formal consent to a contract. Overlaying the relationship is the assumption, on the part of the patient, and a professional commitment, on the part of the health professional, that the latter will provide competent care of the patient's health.

With respect to the legal issues, there are some difference between jurisdictions, with some, such as Australia and the UK, separating the obligation to obtain consent from the related obligation to provide relevant or material information – the duty to inform or to warn. In the US, a doctor who obtains consent but causes harm by treating, without having adequately informed the patient/decision-maker, is more likely to be charged with *trespass to the person* and possibly assault causing actual bodily harm, than in Australia and the UK. In these two countries, if consent has been given but the patient has not been adequately informed about the treatment that caused the harm, then the action would be more likely to be based in *negligence* with respect to the failure to fulfil the duty to inform.

To be ethically valid, consent (or refusal) requires three elements:

- knowledge of relevant information;
- freedom from coercion;
- competence.

Absence of any of these elements may provide some ethical justification for overriding a person's wishes on the basis that, had the person been adequately informed, or not coerced, or competent, he or she would have done otherwise. Obviously this is often the case with children or those who are cognitively impaired, though usually, except in an emergency, consent still needs to be obtained from someone else acting in the person's interests. The view that a person's wishes may be overridden in his or her interests, on the basis that there is such a defect in their decision-making, is called "weak paternalism."[15]

In this respect the ethical practice of medicine is messier than the formal legal concept of consent might imply. However, over the past thirty years the legal requirement to obtain an informed consent before intervening has come to the fore. The duty to provide reasonable care is now likely to be seen as entirely subject to having obtained prior consent. It was not always so. When I first became involved as a hospital ethicist thirty years ago, paternalism and medical authority were the more common emphasis, with much less concern to fully explain the treatment alternatives and the detail of potential complications.

Weak paternalism differs from strong paternalism in that the latter involves a judgement not that there is a defect in the person's decision-making, but rather that the person's judgement is mistaken about his or her own interests, even if adequately informed, free from coercion and competent.

The contemporary notion of respect for autonomy and the internationally recognised right to freedom of thought, conscience and belief, and the rights to privacy and to bodily integrity, would exclude strong paternalism. Weak paternalism is practiced with respect to decisions about a person's competence, and the role of representatives who are required to act in the person's best interests.

1.2.2 The Complexity of Competence

The concept of competence is complex. A person's capacity to make decisions may not be lost even with some cognitive impairment. For instance, a person with dementia may be unable to retain information about the present, limiting the ability to remember having made a decision or to remember information that may bear upon a decision. However the person's understanding of his or her values may

---

15 Ten, Chin Liew, *Mill on Liberty*, Oxford University Press 2001, Chapter 7.

remain intact, leaving the person quite clear about his or her views about a particular treatment option, for instance. It is important not to exclude people with dementia from decision-making, even if they may not remember making a decision.

Competence in an individual can also vary depending on the time of day, the effect of eating or not having eaten, when they take medication, such as blood pressure medication, tiredness, presence of untreated infection such as a urinary tract infection, how much assistance they are given to remember relevant information, and what precisely the nature of the decision may be.

A patient with mild dementia was still driving a car, shopping and cooking for the household and caring for her husband. She was quite competent for most decisions required of her, but on an occasion she was confronted by a draft new will. Her immediate family had wanted her to update to take into account new circumstances. The new will involved complex arrangements for trusteeship for her husband, and disposal of various assets before his death. She was considered by her doctor not to be competent for the purposes of signing the new will. Given her inability to complete a standard memory test, the questions to determine her particular competence for the task of signing the will needed to address whether she did indeed understand the effects of the will and whether it did reflect what she understood her instructions to be in relation to what was to happen after her death. The fact that the draft will completely excluded a son from the will was not part of the intentions she expressed to the doctor and indicated a difference between her understanding and her confusion over the effects of the new draft will. Something like that could happen without malice, just non-trained people not understanding the effects of dementia.

Similarly, the variability of competence in relation to different tasks may be reflected in a person who is alcoholic or drug addicted and unable to make decision in his or her own interest with respect to consumption of the drug perhaps, but competent in relation to other matters such as signing a will.

Competence is thus a notion that may be relative to the matter at hand.

A child or young person's particular level of maturity has implications for whether his or her consent is necessary and/or sufficient. Australia's *National Statement on Ethical Conduct in Human Research* identifies different levels of maturity and the corresponding capacity to be involved in making a decision about participating in research:

A. infants, who are unable to take part in discussion about the research and its effects;
B. young children, who are able to understand some relevant information and take part in limited discussion about the research, but whose consent is not required;
C. young people of developing maturity, who are able to understand the relevant information but whose relative immaturity means that they remain vulnerable. The consent of these young people is required, but is not sufficient to authorise research; and
D. young people who are mature enough to understand and consent, and are not vulnerable through immaturity in ways that warrant additional consent from a parent or guardian.[16]

1.2.3 Representation

Similar considerations may apply in relation to adults with cognitive impairment, depending on the level and nature of the impairment. Often lack of competence and therefore the need to involve a representative in decisions is a complex matter in relation to both timing and the nature of the task. Often it is uncertain and the need is to seek the consent of both the person and their representative to be sure that the right person has provided a competent consent.

---

16 National Health and Medical Research Council, *National Statement on Ethical Conduct in Human Research*, Australian Government 2007, Ch 4.2. http://www.nhmrc.gov.au/publications/ethics/2007_humans/section4.2.htm.

There are several different ways in which someone may become a representative of someone whose competence may be impaired. The representative may be:

- automatically appointed because he or she is the senior available next of kin;
- appointed by a court or tribunal as a guardian or "best friend;" or
- appointed by the patient before he or she became incompetent with an enduring power of attorney for medical treatment.

Depending on the jurisdiction, the person who represents the patient may have a legal obligation to act in that patient's best interests. At time of writing there was a common formula in Australian jurisdictions for determining what that means: in determining a person's best interests, the representative may consider:

- the person's values, beliefs and critical interests;
- the person's previously expressed wishes, to the extent that they can be ascertained, and whether the present circumstances correspond to the situation that the person imagined when expressing or recording those wishes;
- the wishes of a nearest relative or other family members, if it can be confidently assumed that the family's wishes are aligned with the person's interests;
- the benefits and burdens of treatments, and the consequences to the person if the treatment is not carried out, having regard to the level of certainty about prognosis at the time a decision is made;
- the relative merits of any other treatments options;
- the nature and degree of risks associated with the treatment and/or with these options.[17]

---

17 National Health and Medical Research Council, *Ethical Guidelines for the Care of People in Unresponsiveness (Vegetative State) or a Minimally Responsive State* Australian Government 2008.

In the circumstances where the jurisdiction requires a best interests decision, the health professionals involved in the care of a patient have an ethical obligation to seek review of the representation if, in their view, the representative may not be acting in the interests of the patient. The matter is more complicated if the jurisdiction has instead adopted what is often called "substituted judgement", in the place of a best interests determination (see later discussion of representation in Chapter 3.1). Substituted judgement provides the representative with the authority to decide in the place of the represented person and need not reflect acting in their best interests. That person thus holds much greater authority and is less able to be challenged for not acting in the patient's best interests. There is still scope for a concerned health professional, or anyone else, to seek to have a review of the representation, but the grounds are narrower. Basically, to overturn an appointment, they would require evidence that the patient, if competent, would have decided otherwise. The best interests basis of the decision was more open to challenge. The matter is discussed further in the fourth collection of essays in this volume. Still it is important that health professions seek to protect the interests of their patients from negligence, over zealousness or even malice in the representation. Often health professionals in their relationship with the patient may develop a deep understanding of the patient and be motivated by that in deciding to seek review.

As an ethicist, I have on occasion been consulted in aged care circumstances in which, clearly, the representative, a close relative, appeared to want, for various reasons, to get on with life, such as a lady married to a man with dementia in a nursing home, but having met someone else and wanting to be free to pursue her new relationship. Similarly there have been relatives standing to inherit, wanting access to assets sooner rather than later. Substitute consent gives them greater scope and a less challengeable means of refusing non-burdensome care such as flu vaccination or antibiotics that might prolong life and delay the day of inheritance. Health professionals have an obligation to their patient, if they suspect the motives of the representative, to have the representation reviewed, but it is made harder if the jurisdiction has replaced best interests as the criterion with substituted judgement. (See the later extended discussion of representation.)

1.3 Truth-Telling in Health Care

One of the problems that a health professional may face is the extent of the obligation to inform a patient about his or her condition and treatment options. Respect for the truth is important because knowledge is a basic human good. Developing in knowledge is one of the ways in which we flourish. Knowledge is also important because our decisions are based upon it. Deceiving someone or withholding information is a way of manipulating them, and may be coercive.

The way one understands the doctor-patient relationship has a bearing on the way the obligation to inform is interpreted.

When the relationship is understood as *authoritarian or paternalistic*, information may be withheld from the patient on the basis that it would be in the patient's best interests not to know. Thus a health professional may consider that information such as a poor prognosis may cause a patient to give up or lead them to suicide, or may upset them too much.

Within a *free market* understanding of the relationship, it may be seen as the patient's responsibility to find out about the treatment options and whether, for instance, cosmetic surgery is in his or her interests and the record of success of the doctor with like procedures. *Caveat emptor* applies in a free market.

Where the relationship is understood as a *contract,* the understanding of the obligation to inform may depend on the nature of the perceived contract and the obligations it entails. There may be great emphasis on the documentation provided, and the patient may be given considerable detail about the treatment options, as a basis for his or her decision, and little guidance about what the doctor considers to be in the patient's best interests.

Under a *fiduciary model*, the obligation may be shaped by trust that the health professional will act in the patient's best interests. Usually we expect a doctor to inform us of his or her judgement about what is the best treatment option and if there are differing medical views about best practice, what those differences are. In other words, we trust in the competence of the health professional. We also expect to be warned about risks of harm that may affect our decision to accept treatment. In a fiduciary model there may be an understanding that accepts trust in the doctor's decisions and less of an obligation to provide all the relevant information considered necessary in a contractual model. In a fiduciary model the patient may refuse to be given information that he or she does not wish to hear, trusting in the doctor's judgement.

The problem for doctors in warning of risks is to determine how much information to provide and when. Often, complex information needs to be provided to a patient gradually and over time, as it cannot be instantly absorbed. In particular, a prognosis of major or terminal illness may take time for a patient to comprehend and to make adjustments. The immediate reaction may be emotional and may bar further reception of information beyond the bare reality that, for instance, the patient has cancer.

This, however, is not always the way it is done. I recall, a long time ago, discussing with the medical staff at St. Vincent's the issue of information giving. Later I was invited on the ward round accompanying a senior surgeon (with a registrar, the senior nurse and some residents). With the team of us in tow, he approached a patient, following surgical investigation, and said to the patient, "We managed to have a good look at the problem in your gut. I am afraid to say that you are riddled with cancer."

The information may have been an accurate description, but certainly not sensitively delivered. The better practice that I have observed is to focus on what can be done to help as the need for treatment is gradually explained. Asking the patient to explain the diagnosis, prognosis, treatment options and side effects is often very informative about the gaps in knowledge and the need for greater, and perhaps a different style of, information sharing. That then can allow the introduction of revised information about treatment, diagnosis and prognosis.

Australia's National Health and Medical Research Council (NHMRC) writes of informing as a gradual process. The way the doctor gives information should help a patient understand the illness, management options, and the reasons for any intervention. It may be helpful to convey information in more than one session. The NHMRC's recommendations to doctors are:

- Communicate information and opinions in a form the patient should be able to understand.
- Allow the patient sufficient time to make a decision. The patient should be encouraged to reflect on opinions, ask more questions, consult with the family, a friend or advisor. The patient should be assisted in seeking other medical opinion where this is requested.
- Repeat key information to help the patient understand and remember it.
- Give written information or use diagrams, where appropriate, in addition to talking to the patient.
- Pay careful attention to the patient's responses to help identify what has or has not been understood.
- Use a competent interpreter when the patient is not fluent in English.[18]

The difficult question is how much information to give to enable patients to assess, realistically and constructively, the relative risks of a treatment. People may be put off by a long list of possible side effects and adverse reactions of a treatment even though the risks are

---

18 National Health and Medical Research Council, *General Guidelines for Medical Practitioners on Providing Information to Patients*, Australian Government, 1993.

relatively small. Assessing the significance of overall relative risk when there is a multiplicity of low risks is complex. There is a level of risk that we accept in ordinary living. The increased risk associated with medical treatment is balanced against the nature of the symptoms to be treated or prevented and the longer term risks of the disease and there is no formula for that assessment. Many of us rely on medical judgement in that respect.

The legal duty of disclosure has evolved over time, as the doctor-patient relationship has evolved from authoritarian and paternalistic to becoming more fiduciary or contractual on the one hand, and free market, on the other, in some areas of medical practice. The test that used to be applied was the standard of what the reasonable doctor could be expected to do, the so-called "Bolam test" established by Justice McNair[19] in an English case. The case lays down the typical rule for assessing the appropriate standard of reasonable care in negligence cases involving skilled professionals (e.g. doctors). Where the defendant has represented him or herself as having more than average skills and abilities, this test expects standards that must be in accordance with a responsible body of opinion, even if others differ in opinion. In other words, the Bolam test states that *"If a doctor reaches the standard of a responsible body of medical opinion, he is not negligent."*[20]

The Bolam principle was succinctly expressed by Lord Scarman in *Sidaway v. Governors of Bethlem Royal Hospital (1985)*:

> The Bolam principle may be formulated as a rule that a doctor is not negligent if he acts in accordance with a practice accepted at the time as proper by a responsible body of medical opinion even though other doctors adopt a different practice. In short, the law imposes a duty of care: but the standard of care is a matter of medical judgment.[21]

---

19 *Bolam v Friern Hospital Management Committee* (1957) 1 WLR 583.
20 Ibid.
21 House of Lords, *Sidaway vs Bethlem Hospital* (1984) AC 871.

The legal obligation was changed in Australia by a case called *Rogers v. Whitaker*. Ms Whitaker had been almost completely blind in her right eye since a penetrating injury to it at the age of nine. In 1983, almost forty years after her initial injury, she decided to have an eye examination in preparation for a return to the paid workforce. She was referred to Dr Rogers, an ophthalmic surgeon, who advised her that an operation on her right eye would not only improve its appearance but would probably restore significant sight to that eye. The operation was carried out with the appropriate skill and care. However, the surgery did not restore sight in her right eye and, tragically, she also developed sympathetic ophthalmia in her left eye, which resulted in a loss of sight in her left eye. The evidence was that the risk of developing sympathetic ophthalmia was approximately one in 14,000, although the risk of occurrence was slightly greater where there had been an earlier penetrating injury to the eye operated upon (as was the case here). Ms Whitaker had "incessantly" asked questions about possible complications and had inquired as to whether something could have been put over her good eye during the operation.[22]

The High Court eventually said:

> The law should recognise that a doctor has a duty to warn a patient of a material risk inherent in the proposed treatment; a risk is material if, in the circumstances of the particular case, **a reasonable person in the patient's position**, if warned of the risk, would be likely to attach significance to it or if the medical practitioner is or should reasonably be aware that **the particular patient**, if warned of the risk, would be likely to attach significance to it. The duty is subject to the therapeutic privilege.[23] [my emphasis added]

The actual patient test was then modified further by what came to be known as *Woods v. Lowns and Procopis*.[24] The plaintiff in this case

---

22 *Rogers v. Whitaker* (1992) 175 C.L.R. 479, 489.
23 Ibid.
24 *Woods v Lowns and Procopis* (1995) 36 NSWLR 344.

was an eleven year old boy with a history of epilepsy. The plaintiff had been treated by the defendant, Procopis, a paediatric neurologist, from 1979 to 1986. One morning in 1987, the plaintiff's mother went out for a walk and came back to find her son having a fit. She immediately sent her eighteen year old son to get an ambulance and sent her fourteen year old daughter to get a doctor. The daughter ran down to Dr Lowns's surgery, approximately 300 metres away, and told him that her brother was having a bad fit and asked him to help. The doctor declined to attend. When the daughter returned home, the ambulance officers were attempting to treat the boy and rushed the boy to another nearby surgery. The general practitioners there were unable to bring the fit to an end. The boy was then taken to a hospital where the fit was stopped, but by this time he had suffered serious brain damage and remained totally disabled.[25]

The trial judge, Badgery-Parker J, found that Procopis's failure to inform the parents about the use of rectal Valium in emergencies constituted a breach of his duty of care to the plaintiff. Badgery-Parker J also found that if the defendant Lowns had attended to the boy when asked, the appropriate treatment would have commenced seventeen to twenty minutes earlier and the plaintiff would have escaped brain damage.[26]

On appeal, the majority of the Court of Appeal (Kirby P and Mahoney JA, with Cole JA dissenting) reversed the trial judge's findings that Dr Procopis had not satisfied the requisite standard of care. Dr Procopis argued, that unlike Rogers, this case involved treatment rather than advice. However, Kirby P found that the Rogers principle was one of general application, but, nonetheless, he found that this case was better seen as one of advice rather than treatment. There had been substantial agreement in the expert evidence that Dr Procopis's advice conformed with the highest standard of medical practice in Australia. In reversing the trial judge's decision, Kirby P found that limited yet

---

25 Ibid.
26 Ibid.

important use is to be made of normal medical practice. Mahoney J noted that in clinical decisions of this kind the court would be reluctant to put aside the considered opinion of experts in the field.[27]

There is an acceptance that a patient must be informed, if he or she is competent. The legal issues have been about the level or particularity of the information, especially given the complexity of medical decisions. However it still remains the case that there can be obstacles to truth telling. Also, as mentioned earlier, in practice it is not always a neat three stage process of completing the informing of the patient (or representative), obtaining the patient's consent and then commencing treatment. The gradualness of the patient's capacity to understand and the need to begin treatment are likely to involve consent in a state lacking all the material information by whatever standard is applied. Consent may also be implied rather than a formal event and, as discussed earlier, it must remain open to later refusal at any stage, not like contracting to buy a house or car.

The gradualness of the information process aside, the reasons why information may be withheld may be complex. Sometimes in the circumstances of a difficult diagnosis, family members will apply pressure to withhold information on the basis that the patient will "give up" or be otherwise unable to cope with the information. Motivation of that kind may not be restricted to the relatives in relation to the patient. Diagnosis and prognosis can be confronting and there may be fears on behalf of all those involved. If they all know and they know that the others know, then they must face the gravity of the situation. Health professionals can find it difficult to deliver bad news. People can also be resistant to hearing bad news.

The harm done by withholding information includes:

- denying the patient the opportunity to make decisions or even to adjust and to accept death,
- denying the patient time in prospect of death to put affairs in order including making peace with others;

---

27 Lowns & Anor v Woods & Ors (1996) Aust. Torts Reports 81–376, 63,151.

Care of the Sick and the Dying

- denying the relatives that special time in prospect of death to adjust, to repair fractured relationships and to say their farewells while the patient is still functioning;
- fracturing of relationships between those in the know and those who do not; and
- consequent isolation of the patient as some topics become taboo.

One patient I vividly recall was affected in this way. I have made changes to some details to preserve anonymity of participants.

Karlo, a Yugoslav migrant with very little English, had been admitted to hospital for investigation of chronic headache. He was still employed and had no other symptoms. Investigation yielded the diagnosis of a malignant brain tumour. Upon surgical examination it was decided that an attempt to remove the tumour should be made. Following the operation Karlo had lost much of the use of his left side and was virtually immobilized. At the time of the diagnosis, the existence and malignant nature of the tumour had been explained to Karlo's wife and to his adult children, and the family's consent had been obtained to perform the operation after an accurate account of the risks, possible benefits and prognosis had been given to them. Karlo's wife had persuaded the health care team that he should not be told of the cancer. She expressed the opinion that he would lose all hope were he to be told, as a friend of his had died of cancer and he had a great fear of it.

Two years later, Karlo had become isolated as a result of not being told the original diagnosis, as the nurses were unable to discuss it with him. When I saw him he was an angry man who thought that his paralysis was due to a surgical error. To have informed him at that stage of what had happened would have created difficulties for his family, who had persisted in what was in effect a deception. They were locked into the situation by what had occurred initially.

According to the NHMRC, there are ethical issues in:

- how a person's prognosis and likely pathway, and the uncertainty inherent in these predictions, is communicated;
- how differences of opinion are respected and decisions made;

- maintaining a central focus on the person and his or her best interests, throughout a process that is often emotionally difficult as well as ethically complex; and
- who is given information about a person's medical condition.[28]

Effective communication involves:

- identifying families' and other carers' current knowledge, understanding, preparedness to receive information, and information needs at the time;
- sensitivity to the emotional nature of discussion about levels of care;
- respect for patient, carers and family members;
- opportunities for family members and other carers to ask questions and express doubts and concerns;
- use of open-ended questions;
- listening to family members' and other carers' understanding of the person's condition, prospects and care options, their hopes, and their difficulties in providing care and support;
- clarifying any lack of understanding, using terms and concepts that the family and other carers understand; and
- being alert to responses that may indicate denial or blocking of information, and
- responding with care and respect.[29]

Working with Aboriginal and Torres Strait Islander people may involve further complexity including:

- religious beliefs about the person's spirit;
- obligations, respect and responsibilities between family groups;
- additional components of care to be negotiated;

---

28 National Health and Medical Research Council, Op. Cit.
29 Ibid.

- family members staying in the room, especially for younger people;
- sensitive, plain language conversations about the person's condition and options available (prognosis); and
- options for members of the extended family to be involved, to foster trust and greater understanding of the condition.[30]

There is a need to support families by:

- assessing the situation on an ongoing basis;
- seeking and advocating for adequate professional and other support for the family, which may require liaison with government and/or private agencies;
- exploring respite care possibilities and/or possible changes to the site of care, where necessary;
- taking into account the potentially complex effects on families and the person when the condition changes; and
- respecting and seeking to address the family's burden of care with a sufficient level of resourcing and support including psychological care.[31]

1.4 Professional Conscience

The Australian Medical Council (AMC) published ethical guidelines, *Good Medical Practice: A Code of Conduct for Australia's Doctors*,[32] to be applied by Australian Medical Practitioners' Boards, in each State, responsible for maintaining standards in medicine in Australia. Doctors who do not comply can be questioned for their non-compliance and may have their registration to practice restricted

---

30 Ibid.
31 Ibid.
32 Australian Medical Council *Good Medical Practice: A Code of Conduct for Australia's Doctors* (2010) http://www.amc.org.au/images/Final_Code.pdf.

or cancelled. Paul Kommesaroff and Ian Kerridge[33] describe the creeping authoritarianism and the adopting of a narrow ideology by the AMC.

Their concerns are well founded, particularly as the Code indicates a shift away from a Hippocratic approach, that recognises a doctor's professional commitment to serve the health interests of a patient, toward respect for patient autonomy that reduces the health professional to serving patients' needs and expectation. The Hippocratic practice of medicine is made more difficult by the Code as is explained below.

Unfortunately in Australia, neither Federal nor State or Territory law offers protection for freedom of conscience, thought and belief. If anything, the freedom may be in legal jeopardy through the operation of equal opportunity laws which may make it unlawful to withhold service on the conscientious grounds that the provision of the service to a person in given circumstances would be contrary to a health professional's conscientiously held beliefs. For instance, in Victoria, clinicians who provide assisted reproductive technology could be held to be in breach of the Assisted Reproductive Technology Act 2008 if they withheld assistance to achieve pregnancy for a single person or a same sex couple, including a male same sex couple engaging a surrogate, on the conscientious grounds that the child would be deprived of parenting by both a mother and a father.

Until recently, conscientious objection by health professionals was a right that was upheld in practice without recourse to its status or lack of status in State or Federal law. There was respect for the ethical principle that a health professional was entitled to withdraw from providing a service if he or she had a conscientious belief that to do so would be wrong. I have several times been involved in seeking mediation for junior health professionals or those in training who had sought to withdraw from being involved

---

33 Paul A. Komesaroff and Ian Kerridge "The Australian Medical Council draft code of professional conduct: good practice or creeping authoritarianism", *MJA*, Vol. 190 No 4, 16 February 2009, pp. 204-5.

in a particular procedure. For those in training it was important that they could demonstrate that they had the knowledge and skills without actually having to do something that they considered immoral. Thus a gynaecological registrar could demonstrate the ability to do a procedure to do a dilation and curettage to remove a foetus that had died in utero, without having to terminate a viable pregnancy. A neurological registrar could demonstrate the knowledge and capacity to undertake the procedures to assess loss of the clinical indicators for brain stem function without actually having to make or confirm a diagnosis of death by the brain criterion on grounds that he or she did not consider adequate. I am pleased to note that mediation on the basis of conscientious objection, in my experience, has never failed to resolve the issue in favour of the conscientious objector.

The acceptance and understanding of conscientious objection has thus been an admirable quality of senior medical staff and administrators in Australia. However, it is under threat because the ethical acceptance may be shifting and because the ethical respect for the principle that has existed in practice has not been supported by the law. Notably the editor of the *Journal of Medical Ethics,* Dr Julian Savulescu has declared a position opposed to the traditional understanding, arguing amongst other things that it is inefficient and that those who conscientiously object to abortion, particularly, should be excluded from medical practice.[34]

When the *Good Medical Practice* document was issued by the AMC as a draft for public consultation, it contained a concept of "patient-centredness" which was defined in the following way:

> "Patient-centeredness involves perceiving and evaluating health care from the patient's perspective and then adapting care to meet the needs and expectations of the patient."

---

[34] See for instance, Savulescu, Julian. "Conscientious Objection in Medicine." *BMJ* 2006; 332: 294–297; and "Should doctors practice according to their beliefs?" *MJA* 195 (9). 7 November 2011, p. 497.

This sentence left out the normative aspects of a doctor's role which is focussed on what is best for the health of the patient. A patient who is an alcoholic or otherwise addicted or who does not comply with taking needed medication may have perspectives that do not value health or which are irrational with respect to what is in his or her best interests. A patient may demand cosmetic or other non-therapeutic interventions, alternative medicines not based on evidence, or treatment unsuited to his or her condition. The clause would imply that the patient's perspective should override evidence-based professional judgement and the ethical standards of the health professional. It is one thing to respect a patient's right to refuse the advice or the care options offered, it is quite another to demand that the advice and the treatment options be determined, not by the medical evidence and commitment to provide for the patient's health needs on the basis of that evidence, but by whatever perspective the patient has, including perspectives that are well beyond the realm of medical care.

The sentence suggested that the doctor should override considerations of what is in the best interests of the patient's health and simply substitute whatever possibly irrational or unethical judgement the patient may have made as the guide to what the doctor advises or provides. This sentence would seem to have excluded the doctor from giving needed advice in the best interests of the patient's health. It also gives no place for the doctor's own values as a professional committed to serving the health needs of his or her patients. In effect this sentence overturns the Hippocratic tradition and the idea of medicine as a professional vocation. The doctor would cease to be a professional and simply become the most menial of servants, because even servants should have their dignity respected.

The sentence presumably meant to respect the decision-making of the patient, but that respect should not mean that the doctor surrenders his or her own discernment and professional judgement. The trust that a patient has in a health professional is based on the belief the health professional will give advice and offer treatment that best serves the health needs of the patient while respecting the

Care of the Sick and the Dying

patient's right to reject the advice or the treatment offered. The patient need not accept that advice or the treatment offered, but the doctor should be an honest broker in presenting what he or she thinks are the best advice and the best available treatment options to meet the health needs of the patient.

The draft document also asserted:

> "You must ensure that your personal views do not adversely affect your professional relationship with patients."

The draft did not anywhere deal with the issue of conscientious objection, so there was no balance to this requirement and the concept of patient-centredness.

Following public consultation the final document issued had changed significantly in relation to these matters. The concept of patient-centredness was explained in the following way:

> Good medical practice is patient-centred. It involves doctors understanding that each patient is unique, and working in partnership with their patients, adapting what they do to address the needs and reasonable expectations of each patient. This includes cultural awareness: being aware of their own culture and beliefs and respectful of the beliefs and cultures of others, recognising that these cultural differences may impact on the doctor–patient relationship and on the delivery of health services.

Note especially the qualification of the patient's expectations to "reasonable expectations" and accepting that beliefs and culture of the doctor as well as the patient may impact the relationship and the delivery of health services.

Second, a new conscientious objection clause was added:

> 2.46 Being aware of your right to not provide or directly participate in treatments to which you conscientiously object, informing your patients and, if relevant, colleagues, of your objection, and not using your objection to impede access to treatments that are legal.

2.4.7 Not allowing your moral or religious views to deny patients access to medical care, recognising that you are free to decline to personally provide or participate in that care.

Clause 2.46 could have been stronger in addressing the obligation of health professionals to respect the rights of others to conscientiously object and to include a no-disadvantage clause in that respect so that someone who conscientiously objects is not penalised. The right is expressed without acknowledgement of whom it might bind and what their obligations may be. The National Health and Medical Research Council, on the other hand, includes in several of its ethical guidelines a conscientious objection clause that requires other health professionals and health and research institutions to ensure that there is no disadvantage including:

- *National Statement on Ethical Conduct in Human Research* (2007) n. 3.6.7; n. 4.1.14
- *Organ and Tissue Donation after Death, for Transplantation* (2007) n. 2.5
- *Ethical Guidelines on the Use of Assisted Reproductive technology in Clinical Practice and Research* (2007) n. 5.9.

Conscientious objection is only protected when those in authority over another respect the right and create accessible avenues for its exercise. It is much more important to express it as an obligation than as a right.

Second, there is some ambiguity about the issue of referral in the AMC code. This has become an issue in the State of Victoria where the abortion legislation requires doctors who conscientiously object to refer to a doctor who does not conscientiously object (see discussion below). The AMC document appears to provide little protection to a doctor who chooses not to refer for abortion. It protects only not providing or directly participating in treatment to which the doctor conscientiously objects. Referral is not a treatment. Many health practitioners who hold that doing abortion is unethical also regard it as unethical to professionally cooperate in abortion by "referring to another whom the practitioner knows does not have a conscientious objection to abortion". A referral is not a morally neutral act. It implies approval of the conduct and it involves cooperation in the act. For those who hold that abortion is killing a human being, as the Church believes and teaches, clearly, asking them to refer is contrary to conscience.

The Catholic Health Australia *Code of Ethic Standards* states:

> Catholic facilities should not provide or refer for abortion, that is procedures, treatments or medications, whose primary purpose or sole immediate effects is to terminate the life of a foetus or an embryo before or after implantation.

By expressing conscientious objection as a right, but not clearly dealing with the obligations involved on the part of the objector and his or her colleagues and superiors, the AMC code creates some confusion about what conduct is appropriate. Consider the following circumstances:

- a patient requests conduct of a doctor which the doctor considers to be unethical or immoral (e.g. a patient requests termination of pregnancy on the grounds that she would prefer a child of a different gender);
- the doctor is aware that he or she may be asked to undertake or refer for a procedure which is not unlawful but which many members of the profession consider to be unethical or immoral (e.g. surgery to give a healthy fifteen year old girl longer, "more elegant" legs);
- the doctor is aware that while many others consider a particular practice to be acceptable, he or she would find it unethical (e.g. transgender surgery).

The AMC code indicates that the doctor has a "right to not provide or directly participate" in the procedure, but what then? The doctor is obliged not to impede the patient's access to treatments that are legal. Would that mean that the doctor could not, for instance, notify the authorities of a lawful but unethical practice by a colleague to whom the patient sought access, on the grounds that doing so might impede the patient gaining access to the treatment? Suppose for instance that the doctor is aware of a colleague who practices cosmetic surgery lawfully but not very competently and frequently has disastrous results. For the profession to judge the conduct of the colleague only on the grounds of whether it is lawful seems to be a poor standard to apply. In those circumstances it would seem to be proper for the doctor to take what lawful steps he or she could take to impede the patient's access to treatment that may well harm the patient, such as by warning the patient or notifying the medical authorities.

It is laudable that the Australian Medical Council amended the document to include a conscientious objection clause, but more needed to be done to make the clause effective as an obligation on the part of colleagues and those in authority over another health professional.

In the context of framing policy in this area it is important to note that Australia is a signatory to the *International Covenant on Civil and Political Rights*, and therefore has an obligation to protect the right to freedom of thought, conscience and religion:

Article 18

1. Everyone shall have the right to freedom of thought, conscience and religion. This right shall include freedom to have or to adopt a religion or belief of his choice, and freedom, either individually or in community with others and in public or private, to manifest his religion or belief in worship, observance, practice and teaching.
2. No one shall be subject to coercion which would impair his freedom to have or to adopt a religion or belief of his choice.

The AMC document could deal with the religious and political views section simply by saying something like:

Care of the Sick and the Dying 55

> You must avoid exploiting the vulnerability of patients by taking the opportunity to promote causes of a political, commercial, spiritual or religious nature in an unwelcome way.

The document could deal with the conscientious objection issue by saying:

> Where you have a conscientious objection to a particular procedure the patient's health or life must not be endangered and if necessary arrange for care by another practitioner.

And it should require a doctor to respect the conscientious positions taken by colleagues by saying something like:

> Respect the ethical, moral or religious beliefs of medical and other professional colleagues, even if they differ from your own, and their right to practice according to what they perceive are the highest ethical standards.

And could add something about teamwork to the effect:

> Notify the institution and or practice colleagues in a timely manner if you have an ethical objection to a procedure so that other arrangements may be made.
>
> Respect the ethical beliefs of others and do not exercise your right to conscientious objection in a way that implies that the conscientious practice of others is unacceptable.
>
> Where a colleague exercises his or her right to conscientious objection to participate in an activity, respect his or her right to freedom of thought, conscience and religion to do so and do not cause him or her to be disadvantaged on account of that conscientious practice.

This matter could thus be better dealt with by the national AMC guidelines. However that would still leave health professionals without legal protection for freedom of conscience in Australian jurisdictions. The issue is particularly fraught for juniors, those in training and those in subservient positions. The lack of adequate protection may be career ending. In other words the legal and regulatory structure could exclude those who would practice medicine or allied health care Hippocratically, or otherwise implement high ethical standards.

The matter of patient autonomy was discussed extensively in *About Bioethics, volume one: Philosophical and Theological Approaches* so I will not repeat it here. The issue is the use of autonomy as a moral trump overriding respect for the worth of the person, including upholding autonomous choices that would restrict or destroy the capacity to be autonomous. There is a contemporary battle between patient autonomy, as the dominant or only value in health care, and the idea of a health care profession committed to offering the best evidence-based advice and treatment to maintain or restore health, slow the progress of disease and treat uncomfortable distressing symptoms by legitimate, ethical means.

There is a need for legislative protection of conscience within reasonable limits. Unfortunately, in the Australian State of Victoria, the reverse has occurred.

Under Victoria's *Abortion Law Reform Act* 2008, many prolife health practitioners and institutions find that their practices are under threat if they are unwilling to advise or perform an abortion or refer for abortion. The right to conscientious objection by professional health practitioners has been significantly curtailed.

Section 8 of the Act states:

Obligations of registered health practitioner who has conscientious objection

8. Obligations of registered health practitioner who has conscientious objection

1. If a woman requests a registered health practitioner[35] to advise on a proposed abortion, or to perform, direct, authorise or

---

35 Includes medical practitioners, nurses, psychologists and pharmacists.

supervise an abortion for that woman, and the practitioner has a conscientious objection to abortion, the practitioner must-
   a. inform the woman that the practitioner has a conscientious objection to abortion; and
   b. refer the woman to another registered health practitioner in the same regulated health profession who the practitioner knows does not have a conscientious objection to abortion.
2. Subsection (1) does not apply to a practitioner who is under a duty set out in subsection (3) or (4).
3. Despite any conscientious objection to abortion, a registered medical practitioner is under a duty to perform an abortion in an emergency where the abortion is necessary to preserve the life of the pregnant woman.
4. Despite any conscientious objection to abortion, a registered nurse is under a duty to assist a registered medical practitioner in performing an abortion in an emergency where the abortion is necessary to preserve the life of the pregnant woman.

Section 6 of the Act also extends the practice of abortion to permit a registered pharmacist or registered nurse, who is authorised under the **Drugs, Poisons and Controlled Substances Act 1981,** to administer or supply a drug to cause an abortion in a woman who is not more than 24 weeks pregnant.

Section 7 of the Act also allows that a registered nurse or pharmacist may administer or supply a drug to cause an abortion in a woman, who is more than 24 weeks pregnant, if the pharmacist is employed or engaged by a hospital, and at the written direction of a registered medical practitioner.

Doctors, nurses, pharmacists and psychologists would thus have to refer for abortion if they were unwilling to advise or perform an abortion. Catholic institutions that require their health professionals to abide by their code of ethics now have a conflict between their codes of ethics and the legal requirement for health professionals engaged in those institutions to perform or to refer for abortion.

The Victorian Act overturns the age old respect for conscientious exercise of professional judgment, and is at odds with the current inclusion of conscientious objection clauses by the Royal Australian College of Nursing, by the Australian Medical Association and by the National Health and Medical Research Council. The Council not only upholds conscientious objection in its code of ethics, it asserts a no disadvantage clause. For instance, the guidelines on use of foetal tissue in research state:

> 'Those who conscientiously object to being involved in conducting research with separated foetuses or foetal tissue should not be compelled to participate, nor should they be put at a disadvantage because of their objection.'[36]

As mentioned earlier similar, 'no disadvantage' clauses can be found in NHMRC guidelines on organ donation and brain death, assisted reproductive technology (ART), the use of stem cells and medical research.

In relation to psychologists and social workers, the Australian Bishops Conference provided *Advice on Pregnancy Support and Counselling Services (2006)*. In that advice they noted that

> "Decision-making counselling ought not to attempt to direct the patient in relation to her pregnancy or toward any particular decision. The client is most likely to make a good choice if the counsellor serves to reduce the sense of panic and urgency and instead assist the client to regain control of her own circumstances. The aim is to give her greater confidence in being able to cope with pregnancy and to assist her to make a reasonable decision for herself. This provides the best chance of a life-affirming choice."

and the Catholic Bishops went on to say that government funding could not be accepted if it required a counsellor to refer for or actively encourage abortion procedures.

---

36 NHMRC *National Statement on Ethical Conduct in Human Research* Australian Government 2007 n. 4.1.14.

The Victorian Act also requires that despite any conscientious objection a doctor is under a duty to perform an abortion in an emergency where the abortion is necessary to preserve the life of the pregnant woman. This raises questions about whose judgement is to be applied, because there often are alternative ways to manage risks to life and health other than direct abortion. Under the CHA code, loss of foetal life may be permitted when it is not directly intended as a means or an end if there is no other way of saving the woman's life. The Act makes no such distinction.

Nurses have an even worse problem because they would be "under a duty to assist" in a late term abortion, if a doctor requests and claims that it is an emergency. Doctors at least can exercise their discretion and many hold that late term abortion is never medically necessary. Attempting live birth is a safer option if the woman's life is in danger. Late abortion usually involves an additional procedure such as fatal injection to the child in utero. Under the Act nurses are not permitted to object even though doctors can.

When the Act was considered by Parliament, the Scrutiny of Acts and Regulations Committee (SARC) raised a number of concerns about the *Abortion Law Reform Act* 2008. In an Alert Digest to the Parliament it raised several questions about the effect of the Bill on human rights.[37]

However, the Minister's Second Reading Speech remarks included the following:

> In accordance with section 48 of the Charter of Human Rights and Responsibilities, a statement of compatibility for the Abortion Law Reform Bill 2008 is not required. The effect of section 48 is that none of the provisions of the charter affect the Bill. This includes the requirement under section 28 of the charter to prepare and table a compatibility statement, and the obligation under section 32 of the charter to interpret statutory provisions compatibly with human rights under the charter.

---

37 http://www.parliament.vic.gov.au/archive/sarc/Alert_Digests_08/08alt11body.htm#Abortion_Law_Reform_Bill_2008.

Section 48 states:

> Nothing in this Charter affects any law applicable to abortion or child destruction, whether before or after the commencement of Part 2.

As a result it appears from the Hansard that the Parliament did not ever address these questions and the matter of the Bill's incompatibility with the right to freedom of thought, conscience and belief and the rights of human beings before birth.

The Church had not anticipated the interpretation of Clause 48 and had understood that the function of Clause 48 was to prevent judicial opinion using the Charter to broaden the scope of existing abortion law. This opinion was reinforced by the Second Reading Speech for the Charter in which Mr Hulls stated:

> The right to life is a key civil and political right and is protected by the bill. As the provision is not intended to affect abortion laws, a clause is included to put beyond doubt that nothing in the charter affects the law in relation to abortion or the related offence of child destruction. The government is mindful of the range of strong community views on this issue and has never intended the charter, which is aimed at enshrining the generally accepted core civil and political rights, to be used as a vehicle to attempt to change the law in relation to abortion.[38]

Clauses 7 and 8 of the *Abortion Law Reform Act 2008* potentially affect human rights in three areas: freedom of thought, conscience, religion and belief (section 14 of the Charter); the right to hold an opinion without interference (section 15(1) of the Charter); and freedom from compulsory labour (section 11(2) of the Charter).

---

38 Mr Rob Hulls *Second reading Speech, Charter of Human Rights and Responsibilities* Bill 2006 http://www.justice.vic.gov.au/wps/wcm/connect/justlib/DOJ+Internet/resources/4/b/4b6ab080404a3ef9a149fbf5f2791d4a/Second+Reading+Speech.pdf.

In accordance with the Second Reading Speech the Scrutiny of Acts and Regulations Committee also thought that Clause 48 did not prevent the Committee raising questions about the compatibility of the abortion Bill with the *Charter*. In relation to the rights of the child before birth, the Committee found that the Charter provides that 'all persons' have human rights and defines 'person' to mean 'human being'. Overseas courts have held that the question of defining a human being for the purpose of determining the existence of legal rights is a legal (rather than metaphysical or scientific) one and that there is no international consensus on the legal status of foetuses.[39]

The Committee also found that the *Charter* s.7(2) permits all rights to be subject to reasonable limits to further other interests, such as the rights of pregnant women. Overseas courts have held that decriminalisation of abortion can be compatible with foetuses' right to life when accompanied by other adequate measures to discourage abortion, such as state programmes to encourage women to bring pregnancies to term.

During the debate on the Bill, efforts were made to introduce amendments of this kind including:

- Protection for children born alive after an abortion[40]
- Ban on Partial Birth Abortion[41]
- Legal protection (under the Crimes Act) for an unborn child seriously injured during an assault on the mother[42]
- Protection for victims of child sex abuse seeking abortion.
- Information on health risks of abortion[43]
- Independent professional counselling[44]

---

39 http://www.parliament.vic.gov.au/archive/sarc/Alert_Digests_08/08alt11body.htm.
40 Victorian *Hansard* 11 September 2008 p. 3620-3629.
41 Victorian *Hansard* 11 September 2008 p. 3498-3506.
42 Victorian *Hansard* 11 September 2008 p. 3474-3480.
43 Ibid. p. 3629-3631.
44 Ibid. p. 3616.

- Protection for women with disabilities who have impaired decisions-making[45]
- A foetus that is born alive has all the rights of a child[46]
- Approval requirements for abortion clinics[47]
- Offering women 'decision-making' counselling[48]
- Notifying the custodial parent of a child seeking an abortion.[49]
- Keeping an adverse events register[50]
- Requirement to provide foetal tissue samples to police if abuse suspected[51]
- Recording of data on abortion[52]
- Pain relief for foetus[53]

All these amendments were defeated. Section 48 thus created problems by the breadth of the exclusion.

The tragic consequence of the Victorian abortion law is that it has sundered the prior implicit and in practice understanding that health professionals and those in training would be respected if they conscientiously objected and would not be disadvantaged. I have several times had an involvement in the defence of young health professionals for whom that understanding protected them. However the new law showed that this was in fact a challengeable protection which had no basis in Victorian law. The small degree of protection in the Australian Constitution (s. 116) applies only to Commonwealth law. Second, though Australia is a signatory to the International Covenant on Civil and Political Rights (Art 18) that recognises the right to

---

45 Ibid.
46 Ibid.
47 Ibid. p. 3622.
48 Ibid. p. 3536–3550.
49 Ibid. p. 3480–3485.
50 Ibid. p. 3620.
51 Ibid. p. 3619.
52 Ibid. p. 3623.
53 Ibid p. 3625.

Care of the Sick and the Dying 63

freedom of thought, conscience and belief, Australia has not in fact legislated to give effect to its obligation.

That now creates difficulties for health professionals and juniors because the implicit and practical understanding has been shattered. Further, there are those who have applauded the new law for its effects on forcing health professionals to comply with an obligation to refer for abortion against their conscience. The events of 2008 made it much more difficult for people who have conscientious restrictions on what they can do to become trained in medicine, especially gynaecology, and in nursing, pharmacy and psychology, or find and keep employment in those areas. We need legislation to give effect to a no disadvantage conscience clause and to uphold Australia's international obligations to protect freedom of thought, conscience and belief.

1.5 Justice and the Allocation of Scarce Health Resources

Any discussion of the allocation of scarce health resources implies that there is some way of controlling the supply or purchasing of health care services. There are different models in place in different countries and we witnessed a debate in 2010 in the United States over how health care might be managed. The debate took place against a background of the least efficient system in the developed world, and possibly the least efficient health system in the world; in the US, at least 15.2 per cent of gross domestic product is expended on healthcare compared to 9.2 per cent in Australia, 9.9 per cent in Canada, 7.8 per cent in the United Kingdom, 10.4 per cent in France and 10.8 per cent in Germany.[54] At the same time, health care standards are no higher in the US and, in fact, longevity and the average standard of health of the US population are significantly lower than in countries such as Canada and Australia, which have

---

54 Data from Organisation for Economic Co-operation and Development, *OECD Health Data 2006*, from their Internet subscription database, updated October 10, 2006. See http://www.oecd.org/health/healthdata.

universal health care systems.[55] In dialysing when I travel, I am able to make comparisons between health services in different countries, and I am also aware of the comparative data for dialysis patients. Dialysis patients in the US are generally much sicker and have higher mortality than Australian dialysis patients. One of the differences is that American dialysis units tend to rush dialysis sessions, using larger dialysers and taking off fluid at a much greater rate. The motive seems to be cost, but the outcome is much poorer.

Cost and average health standards are a measure of efficiency but not necessarily a measure of justice or fairness. One way to measure fairness is to consider the position of the worst-off. Countries with universal systems such as Australia, England, Germany and Canada, however, do well on that score also.

Some argue that justice is more a matter of liberty than the distribution of goods and services such as health care, and that any attempt to achieve equity in delivery of health care services would violate freedom by requiring government control and restricting those who wish free access to market their goods and services. In discussion with American friends on the comparatively poor state and inefficiency of health care in the US, they are wont to remark to the effect, "But Americans would rather be free than have the alternatives". There is a truth in that, because liberty always upsets attempts to pattern distribution. An efficient, effective health care system might not be achievable, without some level of government control over the provision or purchasing of health services.

In his encyclical *Caritas in Veritate*, Pope Benedict XVI notes that every society draws up its own system of justice. However he teaches that charity goes beyond justice, because to love is to give, to offer what is "mine" to the other; but it never lacks justice, which prompts us to give the other what is "his," what is due to him by reason of his being or his acting. The Pope went on to say,

---

55 Klein, Rudolf "Lessons for (and From) America", *American Journal of Public Health*, January 2003, Volume 93, No. 1, pp. 61–3.

Justice is the primary way of charity or, in Paul VI's words, "the minimum measure" of it, an integral part of the love "in deed and in truth" (1 Jn 3:18), to which St. John exhorts us. On the one hand, charity demands justice: recognition and respect for the legitimate rights of individuals and peoples. It strives to build the *earthly city* according to law and justice. On the other hand, charity transcends justice and completes it in the logic of giving and forgiving. The *earthly city* is promoted not merely by relationships of rights and duties, but to an even greater and more fundamental extent by relationships of gratuitousness, mercy and communion. Charity always manifests God's love in human relationships as well, it gives theological and salvific value to all commitment for justice in the world.[56]

The delivery of health services is owed to those who are sick and in need, but their needs also call us to respond not simply out of duty, but out of love. Our first objective in health care must be to ensure that those in need are humanly cared for. That is not a need for high technology, though technology is certainly a great good, but a need for the warm presence of another who cares and who, by empathy alone, can reduce the burden of illness and suffering. That is so because a significant part of suffering associated with illness is existential. It is to do with loss of status, capacity, isolation and fear (see section five). The only real cure for existential suffering is love. It is a basic requirement of justice that whatever system we have, it must provide at least basic care for those who are sick and in need. No-one should have to die alone. No-one in need of care should be denied it.

It helps to consider what we mean by "health." A simple definition might be the absence of ill-health or disease, or the normal psychosomatic functioning of the organism.

As discussed earlier, the World Health Organisation (WHO) defines health as "a state of complete physical, mental, and social well-being and not merely the absence of disease and infirmity."

---

56 Pope Benedict XVI, *Caritas in Veritate*, Vatican City 2009.

Many have criticised this for including well-being, as well-being equates with happiness and involves much more than is normally meant by health. Well-being includes successful and satisfying exercise of intelligence, awareness, imagination, taste, prudence, good sense, and fellow-feeling.[57]

The problems generated by such a wide definition are inappropriate diagnosis of illness, such that social non-conformity becomes an illness. Health care efforts are misdirected, with over-medicalisation and unreal expectations, such as we have seen with the medicalisation of classrooms by the apparent over-diagnosis of ADHD, the over-management and institutionalization of death and dying, and the overuse of antibiotics.

Healthcare can be defined, less controversially, as intervention that seeks to restore, maintain, or promote health, to prevent or slow the progress of disease, or to alleviate distressing symptoms of ill-health. Healthcare professional intervention and personal health care.

The allocation of resources for healthcare happens at several levels:

- macro-allocation – the proportion of community resources to be devoted to healthcare;
- meso-allocation – the kinds of services to be provided with these resources;
- micro-allocation – who should get the health services provided.

Macro-allocation may be criticised for underspending and misdistribution of needed services, as demonstrated by queuing. Queuing is a form of rationing. Macro-allocation may also be criticised for overspending relative to other social goods such as education, housing, water, nutrition and security. In many parts of the world the greatest barrier to good health is lack of clean water and sanitation. There may also be a concentration on high technology rather than on basic care and primary care, including prevention.

---

57 Kilner, John, *Who Lives? Who Dies? Ethical Criteria in Patient Selection*, YUP, 1984.

Criticisms of meso-allocation may include overspending on;

- crisis, rescue or acute care;
- high technology care;
- institutional care;
- established care rather than research;
- fashionable or traditional care rather than alternatives;
- particular regions – city not rural;
- acute at the expense of chronic illness;
- areas with media and political clout.

Criticisms of micro-allocation may include:

- unjust discrimination on the basis of a person's age, race, gender, disability or disadvantage;
- overspending on those who are articulate and demanding.

Health care has, in recent times, tended to be viewed in utilitarian terms. Rather than focussing on basic care for all those in need and measuring fairness by the situation of the worst off, a utilitarian approach judges a system by utility – the net sum of benefits and losses in terms of maximizing the average or total utility. Such judgements depend on having a way to measure the relative utility of proposals.[58]

One such system involves assessing quality adjusted life years or QALYs. A treatment may then be assigned a value according to predicted quality of life of the patient multiplied by the number of years of life expectancy. The problem with using QALYS is that the judgement about the "quality of life" is problematic and would seem to discriminate against those who are chronically ill or disabled. Someone who is chronically ill does not get better. Hence resources are used simply to maintain him or her. The person scores

---

58 Smart, JJC, "An Outline of a System of Utilitarianism Ethics," Ch 4 in Bernard Williams, *Utilitarian: for and against*, Cambridge University Press 1973.

very badly as an inefficient use of resources, compared to a well person who only needs a short period of treatment to restore health and function.

In the US State of Oregon an attempt was made to ration healthcare on the basis of a psychometric index of quality.[59] The scheme initially attempted to rank conditions and the effects of treatment on a scale of importance. The first attempt was done on the basis of a phone survey and public hearings. There were many anomalies, for example:

- Cosmetic surgery ranked as more important than treating an open fracture of the femur.
- Teeth repair ranked as more important than treating Hodgkin's disease.
- Infertility treatment ranked as more important than obstetric care.

In Oregon Phase Two, they tried to categorise treatments in terms of

- essential services
- very important services
- services valuable to certain individuals
- acute fatal, prevents death
- maternity, neonatal and paediatric
- chronic fatal – improves well-being
- contraception, sterilization
- comfort care – palliation
- preventive care – screening.[60]

---

[59] Sabik, Lindsay M and Lie, Reidar K, "Priority setting in health care: Lessons from the experiences of eight countries", *International Journal for Equity in Health* 2008, Vol 7, No. 4.

[60] Ibid.

It is worth noting that Oregon was the first US State to legalise physician-assisted suicide. One wonders whether that was a result of rationing provoking fear of neglect.

The health care debate over justice often involves a conflict between fee-for-service models and managed care.

Fee-for-service limits the capacity of governments to ration health care and thus control health expenditure, but it protects the autonomy of health professionals to determine what level of care is appropriate and preserves doctor-patient relationships without the interference of another, though the latter can happen through health insurance companies capping expenditure and placing other limits on the care provided.

Managed care involves the establishment of health maintenance organizations in which individuals enrol and the organization buys services from health care providers. This is a way to achieve effective rationing at macro and meso level. It can involve injustices to particular individuals at micro level, especially the chronically ill and others such as those who have mental illness or cognitive disability, lack the local language, lack family supports, are drug users or are homeless. People in all of these situations have complex health needs and require more resources to treat.

All systems have problems of fairness. The important issue is the capacity of a system to make adjustments so that no-one is denied basic care and that higher levels of care are allocated on the basis of need. Healthcare is a relationship between the provider and the person in need, built on the requirements of justice and the need for love. Funding and allocation systems need to protect that human relationship.

As our populations age, there is concern that there will be too few people working to support those who have retired. This is one of the consequences of declining fertility, with most Western nations below replacement level. As the problem increases, it is important that we continue to advocate for the needs of the frail elderly and maintain respect for them. The commandment that we honour our father and our mother has never been so crucial. Economic need now requires families to have two incomes and so few are able to care for their ageing relatives once they need constant attention. It is a great sadness that so many aged people must rely exclusively on care by strangers. There is a need to make better provision for people who would care for their relatives if the economic circumstances permitted it. Funding for caregivers in Australia has prohibitive eligibility requirements and it is not a substitute for a wage.

For many families, often the turning point is when an elderly relative suffers from dementia or becomes incontinent. Dementia can mean the person needs constant attention both for safety reasons and also because dementia can cause loneliness if the person cannot remember recent events like contact with family members and friends. It is not uncommon for a person with dementia to forget, and then complain about being ignored and isolated, despite just having been in company. Without constant attention, dementia can cause great misery. For many contemporary families such attention is not possible, especially if there are children and others also demanding attention. The choice may be between caring for the older person in a state lacking adequate attention and thus a state of poor safety and loneliness, or seeking institutional care for occasional respite, or indefinitely. The choice is often difficult and painful because of the heartfelt attitude that one should be able to care for one's parents and the obligation to honour them. However, institutional care may be in the interests of an older person, if the alternative cannot provide adequate attention to meet safety and the greater social needs, or the burden of so doing is overly demanding and causes overly stressed relationships, and significant unmet needs elsewhere.

Through institutional care the family may also lose the presence of grandparents, the richness they bring and the experience of caring for them. Seeking institutional care does need to be balanced by finding ways and time to include older members in the family and family events, even if most of the care is provided elsewhere.

2. Care ... Until the End

2.1 Care of the Dying and Proportionate Means

When a person is considered to be in the last phase of life, then more than ever, it seems, issues to do with the meaning of life and the purpose for our existence come to the fore. Dying is a most important phase of life, as we are led through growing disability to surrender the things of this life and to prepare for the life to come. Christians believe that it is not an end but a transition to a new beginning.

In the dying process, not only the dying person, but those around them become acutely aware of the human condition. Christians believe that we are essentially made in the image and likeness of God for the purpose of communion with him, and that we are made with free will. We accept the biblical story of mankind in which we are affected by sin, and that our fallen nature is marked by suffering, war, oppression, poverty, vain striving, disappointment and death. Death is part of the human condition: we are born dying – "the wages of sin" (*Rom* 6:23, cf *Gen* 2:17).

At the same time, however, we believe that we are redeemed by Christ's life, death and resurrection and called to communion with him.

That belief in resurrection humanises the dying process by giving us hope. It humanises the dying process by allowing us to accept that life is in transition, that we are called to be with God, and therefore death is both tragedy and gain. Before us, we have the example of Christ who, in prospect of his own death at Gethsemane, expressed his complete and free submission to the will of the Father. His death transformed us through the sacrifice he made for our sins. For us, then, death is the end of our earthly pilgrimage in which we look forward to life in complete communion with him. For that reason, we are not obliged to use every possible means to prolong life but can accept death's inevitability in prospect of the life to come.

Christ's suffering, death and resurrection also provides insight into the mystery of suffering. We know from experience, and from the biblical account of the Fall, that suffering is an inescapable burden of human existence. Christ has also shown that suffering in others provides the opportunity to love as he did, in response to those he encountered. Christ's own suffering also shows us how best to respond in acceptance of the divine will for us. His suffering, especially his cry of abandonment on the Cross, also indicates the human reality of extreme suffering both in its effect on us, which disables rational function, and in our need for the support of others. Empathy diminishes suffering (see Chapter Five).

The experience of suffering is a factor in personal growth: our love of others increases our capacity to suffer, and that love responds effectively to suffering through empathy. We also come to realise that suffering dehumanises, and love humanises both victim and carer. (See Chapter Five).

The Catholic Catechism teaches that life and physical health are precious gifts entrusted to us by God. We must take reasonable care of them, taking into account the needs of others and the common good.[1]

The Catechism also teaches that though morality requires respect for the life of the body, it does not make it an absolute value. It rejects a neo-pagan notion that promotes a *cult of the body*, sacrificing everything for its sake and idolizing physical perfection and success at sports. By preferring the strong over the weak, this can pervert human relationships.[2]

Instead, the Catholic tradition teaches that everyone is responsible for his or her life before God who has given it. It is God who remains the sovereign master of life. We are obliged to accept life gratefully and preserve it for his honour and the salvation of our souls. We are

---

[1] *Catechism of the Catholic Church* St Paul's Publications, 1994, n. 2288.
[2] Ibid. n. 2289.

stewards, not owners, of the life God has entrusted to us. It is not ours to dispose of.[3]

Suicide contradicts the natural inclination of the human being to preserve and perpetuate his or her life. It is contrary to the love of self. It likewise offends love of neighbour because it unjustly breaks the ties of solidarity with family, nation, and other human societies to which we continue to have obligations. In addition, for believers, suicide is contrary to love for the living God because we are made in God's image and likeness.[4]

Discontinuing medical procedures that are burdensome, dangerous, extraordinary, or disproportionate to the expected outcome can be legitimate; it is the refusal of "over-zealous" treatment. Here one does not will to cause death; one's inability to impede it without imposing too great a burden is merely accepted. The decisions should be made by the patient if he or she is competent and able, or, if not, by those legally entitled to act for the patient, whose reasonable will and legitimate interests must always be respected.[5]

Certainly there is a moral obligation to care for oneself, and to allow oneself to be cared for, but this duty must take account of concrete circumstances. It needs to be determined whether the means of treatment available are objectively proportionate to the prospects for improvement. To forego extraordinary or disproportionate means is not the equivalent of suicide or euthanasia; it rather expresses acceptance of the human condition in the face of death.

This distinction predates modern medicine, health insurance and universal public health care systems. It used to be called the distinction between *ordinary and extraordinary means*. It meant that a family should do what a family ordinarily could do to care for a dying person, freeing them of obligations to take extraordinary means, those things that were beyond what a family could ordinarily provide. They were not obliged to provide expensive, difficult professional intervention.

---

3 Ibid. n. 2280.
4 Ibid. n. 2281.
5 Ibid. n. 2278.

Possibly the earliest recording of the distinction was in the writing of a Spanish sixteenth century theologian, Francisco De Vitoria, in his seminal work *Relectiones Theologicae*,[6] where he distinguished between natural means of preserving life – food, rest, etc., and the limited therapeutic interventions of the time.

Another sixteenth century theologian, Domingo Soto, made a similar distinction when he wrote in relation to battlefield amputations (well before the time of general anaesthesia):

> Given that in the amputation of a limb or in cutting open the body there is very great pain, certainly nobody can be obliged to undergo this because nobody is held to preserve their life with so much torment. Nor should that person be deemed someone who commits suicide.[7]

In recent times that distinction has come to mean:

- Ordinary – all interventions that offer a reasonable hope of benefit for the patient and can be obtained and used without excessive expense, pain, or other inconvenience.
- Extraordinary – all interventions that cannot be obtained or used without excessive expense, pain, or other inconvenience for the patient or for others or which, if used, would not offer reasonable hope of benefit for the patient.

The notion of "burdensome treatment" has been explained through the use of examples to include treatment that is: painful, frightening, hazardous, repugnant, disruptive for the patient, repugnant, financially too burdensome to the patient, family, hospital or health service, or would require the use of facilities that are urgently needed by other patients who would benefit more.

---

6 Cf. Clark, Peter, "Tube Feedings and Persistent Vegetative State Patients: Ordinary or Extraordinary Means?", *Christian Bioethics*, Volume 12, No. 1, May 2006 pp. 43–64.

7 Ibid.

The following are some examples (note that the names and other details have been altered so that the examples do not represent any real person), where the distinction applies:

- Mrs Attwood, 85, has had a brain tumour surgically removed but is left with some brain damage including the area that processes olfactory sensation. She complains that all food tastes and smells utterly repugnant to her, "like vaseline." She asks her priest whether she is obliged to keep eating when it is so repugnant to her.
- Mr. Heine, 88, is a survivor of Nazi concentration camp medical experiments. He is a diabetic and has a lesion on his foot that has become infected and is gangrenous and he has developed septicaemia. Amputation of the limb below the knee is recommended as a life-saving measure. He refuses. Part of his refusal seems to be linked to a fear of doctors from his earlier experience, part is repugnance at the thought of losing the limb.
- Mr. Arthurs of Nullawil in the Mallee region of Victoria (Australia) has a prostate malignancy and has started chemotherapy to be followed by radiotherapy. His wife has advanced ischaemic heart disease and can no longer make the 700 kilometre round trip (3.5 hours each way) to Melbourne with him. He asks whether he can refuse the treatment so that he can stay home to look after his wife through her last illness. He does not want to be away when she dies and judges that the burden for her in being without him for long periods would be too great.
- Mr. Multugera, 68, of the Jagara (Australian indigenous) people has lived all his life in the East Kimberley region of Australia. He is an artist and had a missionary school education, but has led a tribal existence isolated from most aspects of modern industrialised society. A tribal elder, he has never visited a settlement of more than a few hundred people. He has been brought into a clinic to see the visiting doctor who comes once a month. He has episodes of chest pain, sweating and weakness. A cardiograph shows evidence of advanced heart disease warranting an

angiogram and probably open heart surgery or a heart transplant. This can only be done by sending him by air ambulance to a major centre such as Perth or Adelaide. This would take him out of his family, tribal and cultural context and he refuses to go.
- Greg is a long-term prisoner with a history of violence that has continued in prison. He has frequently self-mutilated. On one occasion he cut-off his penis. Psychiatric assessment holds that he is not mentally ill so he has remained in an ordinary prison. The Prison Reform Society has lobbied strongly for surgical restoration of his penis. Plastic surgeons judge that he would not be compliant through the long series of operations and rehabilitation, and so indicate that it would not be appropriate as there is little prospect of long-term benefit.
- Mary has been on dialysis for eighteen years. Recently she has developed ischaemic heart disease and as a result she suffers from severe angina for the duration of each dialysis session of five hours, three times per week. Initially she was treated with analgesics but there is a limited range available to those on dialysis because most have metabolites that are not removed by the dialysis and she has now become tolerant of those that she can take to the point that there is no available means of controlling her pain while on dialysis short of general anaesthesia. That is considered inappropriate on such a frequent basis. She has informed her doctor that the treatment has become too burdensome and opts not to continue.

2.2 Not for Resuscitation Orders[8]

Resuscitation generally refers to a set of interventions following cardiac or respiratory arrest including: clearing an obstructed airway, intubation into the airway, defibrillation using an electric shock to restart the heart or to restore its rhythm, adrenaline to stimulate the

---

8 Much of the following reflects the *Not for Resuscitation Policy* that was developed at St. Vincent's Hospital, Melbourne in 1988–9.

heart, cardiac massage to both restart the heart and to compress the lungs to assist breathing, and the administration of a large dose of valium so that the patient does not remember the awful experience, particularly of defibrillation. In a hospital they may then attach a ventilator to the respiratory tube. Out of hospital, the paramedics may use a bag to do the same task.

The issues involved in making decisions about care for the dying are included in section 2.1 "Care of the Dying and Proportionate Means." Decisions on resuscitation are often made ahead of time by issuing a not-for-resuscitation (NFR) order.

Contrary to the soap opera dramas, most attempts to resuscitate do not succeed. Success is most likely following cardiac arrest during or after surgery, or after a trauma such as a knock to the head or drowning. However, when a person arrests as a result of a disease process such as metastatic cancer or advanced heart disease, it is most unlikely that resuscitation will succeed.[9] It is normal practice therefore to regard resuscitation in the circumstances of severe disease as futile and to issue an NFR order when it is judged that the disease process will soon result in death.

The alternative is to attempt resuscitation every time someone dies and no-one would be permitted to die in peace. NFR orders are important for nurses so that they know when not to initiate resuscitation or when not to call an ambulance to a nursing home. Nursing homes are usually not equipped to resuscitate, other than to administer oxygen and first aid measures, including clearing a blocked airway.

---

9 Note that a 2006 review was conducted of forty-two studies from 1966–2005, comprising 1707 patients meeting minimal inclusion criteria. Overall survival to discharge was 6.2%. Survival in patients with localized disease was 9.5%, and in patients with metastatic disease was 5.6%. Analysis of data reported since 1990 reveals a narrowing of the survival gap, with survival rates in patients with localised disease of 9.1%, and in patients with metastatic disease of 7.8%. Survival in patients resuscitated on the general medical/surgical wards was 10.1%, while survival in patients resuscitated on intensive care units (ICUs) was 2.2%. C.f. Reisfield GM, Wallace SK, Munsell MF, Webb FJ, Alvarez ER, Wilson GR. "Survival in cancer patients undergoing in-hospital cardiopulmonary resuscitation: a meta-analysis" *Resuscitation*. 2006 Nov;71(2):152–60, 2006 Sep 20.

Resuscitation is very intrusive. Cardiac massage often breaks ribs, particularly in the frail elderly. Intubation is never comfortable for a person who is conscious, and defibrillation is something nobody would want to experience while at all conscious. Thus resuscitation may be deemed to be overly burdensome for some who are very frail, and an NFR order will be made for that reason even though resuscitation might not be futile.

Some people who have experienced resuscitation for respiratory failure (e.g. those with a neurological condition that predisposes them to it) will insist that in the future they do not want resuscitation to be attempted. An NFR order may then be issued. Deciding that a treatment is overly burdensome is a patient's moral and legal right.

An NFR order applies only to resuscitation. It should never be a death sentence in which all forms of life-prolonging care are withdrawn. Ordinary or relatively non-burdensome treatments such as antibiotics for infection or tube feeding should normally be continued. Nor should an NFR order preclude ordinary assistance for a temporary problem, such as clearing a blocked airway after a person has choked on food.

The issues involved in making NFR decisions can be divided into three categories: indications, consultation and documentation. An NFR order may be issued when:

A. a patient of sound mind and free of any suicidal ideation or temporary depression, and in possession of the relevant medical information about his or her condition, makes a competent decision, free from any coercion by others, to refuse resuscitative interventions that he or she would consider to be overly burdensome or futile (unlikely to succeed), were he or she to arrest;
B. the patient's legally recognised representative for medical treatment decisions, in possession of the relevant medical information about the patient's condition, has reasonable grounds for believing that the patient, if competent, would refuse resuscitative interventions on the grounds that they would be overly burdensome or futile were he or she to arrest; or

Care of the Sick and the Dying   79

C. the patient's doctor judges that the patient's condition is such that, in the event of an arrest, attempts to resuscitate would be futile or would in themselves be overly burdensome for the person.

In making an NFR order, the patient's doctor should consult the patient (if possible), the patient's legally recognised representative for medical treatment, (see chapter three) or in the latter's absence, his or her family and carers. (Many jurisdictions give an automatic legal status to the senior available next of kin.)

To be valid, an NFR order should contain the following information:

A. date of the order;
B. date for review of the order (no more than six months);
C. those consulted (including the patient, if competent, or the patient's legal representative for medical treatment if there is one);
D. the indication for issuing an NFR order;
E. treatment to be continued (eg. clearing blocked airways, oxygen, medication for existing conditions such as antibiotics);
F. specific resuscitative measures to be withheld (eg. calling an ambulance for full-scale para-medical resuscitation or attempting cardiac massage or intubation);
G. doctor's signature and contact details.

2.3   Tube Feeding

Tube feeding, where a tube is placed into the stomach, either

- directly through the wall of the abdomen (percutaneous endoscopic gastrostomy or PEG), or
- via a tube placed through the nose and down into the oesophagus and stomach (naso-gastric tube),

is used for patients who are unable to swallow. In those circumstances the food given is of a fluid consistency like infant formula.

Generally a PEG is considered less of a problem than a nasogastric tube, which can be persistently uncomfortable. Over the past twenty years, with the advent of better methods of placing the tube, softer, more flexible materials for the manufacture of the tube, and better knowledge about avoiding complications, PEG feeding has become much more common. The initial placement of the tube is a surgical procedure but after that, provided no complications develop, feeding usually becomes routine and can be managed at home by people who lack nursing training. Family members often manage it without assistance for very long periods. They simply fill a large-bore syringe with a measured amount of the formula, open the plastic tube into the stomach, and inject the contents of the syringe into the tube. It is important that the person is sitting up, during and after feeding, to avoid the risk of fluid finding its way into the trachea and lungs. The latter may cause respiratory problems, including pneumonia and death.

For patients who have had their bowel removed, a tube may be placed directly into a major blood vessel and nutrients are added to a saline infusion directly into the bloodstream (called total parenteral nutrition – TPN). Because the infusion is not absorbed through the gut, great care must be taken to manage the balance of nutrients in the blood stream and TPN thus requires expensive monitoring with frequent pathology tests. Thus, while TPN can be managed by people who carry on a normal work routine, it does require frequent attendance at a clinic.

When the condition of a person on tube feeding deteriorates, the question may be asked whether to continue with the feeding. Similarly, for people with a severe illness from which there is little possibility of significant recovery (e.g. advanced metastasized cancer, advanced ischaemic heart disease, severe stroke, advanced Parkinson's disease, severe dementia), when they are no longer able to swallow food, the question may be asked whether it is necessary or appropriate to initiate tube feeding.

Without nutrition and hydration, a patient will certainly die, so the question has grave implications.

Generally, the Church has taught that there should be a presumption in favour of providing life-sustaining measures to all patients, including tube feeding,[10] unless the method of delivery is considered to be overly burdensome or futile.[11]

Tube feeding can be considered overly burdensome if problems develop; for example, some people may find a naso-gastric tube to be very uncomfortable, or a person with a PEG may develop chronic inflammation of the lining of the stomach and or the gut, or may repeatedly aspirate food into the trachea and lungs, causing severe respiratory distress.

Tube feeding can also be considered futile if the person develops severe renal impairment or severe ischaemic heart disease, or his or her system is shutting down for other reasons. In such circumstances, continuing to provide hydration may overload the patient's system and cause a more rapid death. Initiating tube feeding may also be considered futile when the patient's condition is so close to death that the feeding will not sustain the life. This is often thought to be the case when a patient reaches such an advanced stage of dementia that he or she can no longer swallow; death is likely to happen soon and feeding will therefore not sustain the life significantly.

When tube feeding is thus futile or overly burdensome, initiating or continuing it is not considered to be obligatory.[12]

When a person requires tube feeding because a stroke or other severe damage to the brain has prevented them from swallowing, it is unlikely that tube feeding would be overly burdensome. The condition

---

10 Pope John Paul II, An address to an International Congress on "Life-Sustaining Treatments and Vegetative State: Scientific Advances and Ethical Dilemmas", Rome Saturday, 20 March 2004 Accessed from: http://www.vatican.va/holy_father/john_paul_ii/speeches/2004/march/documents/hf_jp-ii_spe_20040320_congress-fiamc_en.html.

11 See the discussion of these terms in the section 2.1 of this collection headed "Care of the Dying and Proportionate Means".

12 Ibid.

often becomes relatively stable and some recovery can seldom be totally excluded, although it may be slow.

However the feeding may serve to maintain someone who is in a severely damaged state with poor prospects of a return to health. Often the question is asked whether such a condition is itself futile and the treatment should therefore be withdrawn.

Pope John Paul II addressed this issue:

> I feel the duty to reaffirm strongly that the intrinsic value and personal dignity of every human being do not change, no matter what the concrete circumstances of his or her life. *A man, even if seriously ill or disabled in the exercise of his highest functions, is and always will be a man*, and he will never become a "vegetable" or an "animal".
>
> Even our brothers and sisters who find themselves in the clinical condition of a "vegetative state" retain their human dignity in all its fullness. The loving gaze of God the Father continues to fall upon them, acknowledging them as his sons and daughters, especially in need of help.[13]

Simply expressed, people who are in an unresponsive state or have suffered severe brain damage remain as members of the human family; they remain someone's son or daughter, mother or father, sister or brother. Respect for their lives remains inherent, because it is based not on their contribution, but on who they are. As discussed earlier, and in volume one, all human beings are considered to be of equal dignity, no matter their level of ability or disability.

Reasoning in this way, Pope John Paul II held that the fact that a person remains unresponsive after emerging from coma, and irrespective of how long the patient remains in this state, does not mean that the person is any less deserving of medical treatment and nonmedical care. Such patients should not be abandoned, nor denied ordinary care and life-sustaining measures. In all cases, the judgments

---

13 Pope John Paul II Address to an International Congress on Life Sustaining Treatment and the Vegetative State Saturday, 20 March 2004 *http://www.vatican.va/holy_father/john_paul_ii/speeches/2004/march/documents/hf_jp-ii_spe_20040320_congress-fiamc_en.html.*

about the care due to patients should be based on the relevant medical and ethical criteria, not on the so-called "quality" of the patient's life or state of consciousness.[14]

In the case of feeding, there is often a difference between withholding and withdrawing treatment because there is greater burden in initiating feeding than simply continuing servicing a feeding tube that has already been inserted. To start PEG feeding requires a surgical procedure to create the access, and while the risk associated with the procedure is considered minimal, it is nevertheless a surgical procedure with some attendant discomfort. Further, a very ill patient may be at too high a risk of dying from the anaesthesia. Therefore there can be circumstances in which tube feeding would not be undertaken in someone whose condition is deteriorating and for whom the surgery to initiate tube feeding would be considered too burdensome, given that it is not already in place.

An aspect to consider in decisions about tube feeding is the importance that feeding someone has in our relationship to them. The process of cooking and providing a meal for someone is usually an act of love and expressive of the relationship between people. Tube feeding still has that significance of an act of love, though it can be less meaningful because there is no direct enjoyment, no eating and tasting and associated social events, and the process may be mechanical. Nevertheless, continuing to feed retains the significance of maintaining someone. No-one can live without it. My experience of the circumstances when a decision was made to cease feeding, was that often the relatives received the decision emotionally as giving up, and sometimes they stopped or reduced their visiting at this point. It was as though the decision not to feed meant that their relative might as well be dead, because he or she would be so very soon. Loss of feeding can thus mean loss of supportive relationships. The presumption in favour of continuing feeding is very important for the meaning attached to continuing to support someone.

---

14 Op. Cit.

There has been an unfortunate trend toward using tube feeding, not because a person cannot swallow, but because he or she cannot feed him or herself. Tube feeding is quick and easy, and saves time for staff or family. Spoon-feeding someone who cannot feed themselves is much more labour intensive and thus relatively expensive. This is often an unfortunate casualty of economic rationalism with spoon-feeding replaced by a PEG in patients who can swallow. Sadly, people who are fed by a tube lack the opportunity to enjoy the taste of the food. Even more significantly, servicing the tube can be such a very swift business, and done so impersonally, that they also miss the social communication and the expressions of friendship that often accompany the rituals of eating and drinking. In 1996 when the Victorian government introduced *case-mix funding*, which funded by diagnosis, and then made little allowance for different nursing needs, such as this, the number of patients who had PEGs in place reportedly increased 85%, because of the economic advantage over labour-intensive spoon-feeding.

That is a sad indictment of the policy, for its effect on people no longer permitted to taste and eat and enjoy the social interaction of feeding, even though they could still swallow safely.

I have suggested that if ever that PEG feeding is my circumstance, they might at least use a single malt for mouth hygiene.

2.4 Refusal of Food and Water[15]

2.4.1 Introduction

A number of highly publicised cases in Australia and New Zealand have once again drawn attention to the ethical and legal dilemmas surrounding the provision and refusal of nutrition and hydration at the end of life. Two recent cases that come most readily

---

15 The section was published as Nicholas Tonti-Filippini, 'Further Considerations in Relation to Refusal of Nutrition and Hydration", *Nathaniel Centre Report,* Issue 30, June 2010.

to mind are those of Christian Rossiter, a 49-year-old Perth man who became a quadriplegic in March 2008, and Margaret Page, a 60-year-old Wellington woman who suffered a cerebral haemorrhage 20 years ago.

The cases have a number of similarities: both people wanted to be able to exercise a personal choice about whether or not they continued to live; neither was suffering a terminal illness, nor were they dying – at the time of the debate there was no specific reason to think that either could not have continued to live for a good number of years.

There are, however, significant moral differences. Mr Rossiter relied on artificial nutrition and hydration, while Mrs Page was able to take food and water in the normal way, although she relied on carer support to do that. Mr Rossiter was unable to exercise his personal choice to refuse nutrition and hydration without a mandate from an Australian court; while the Supreme Court of Western Australia affirmed his right to instruct his carers to discontinue his nutrition and hydration, he chose not to exercise this right and eventually died from pneumonia in September 2009. Meanwhile, in New Zealand, Mrs Page's decision to refuse food and water was judged by most as the right of any competent person upheld by section 11 of the New Zealand Bill of Rights. Mrs Page died of the effects of starvation in March 2010.

These two cases have stimulated renewed discussion in Catholic circles. The following sections raise a number of questions that follow from a person's decision to refuse nutrition and hydration; questions that have, by and large, not been well aired in the coverage of these and other similar cases. They are particularly relevant for staff and management of Catholic health-care facilities.

2.4.2 Gaps in the Discussion

I support the conclusion that a Catholic facility should not refuse to care for someone in the circumstances of the Christian Rossiter case in Western Australia, but the matter is much more complicated than some suggest. It is also my view that a Catholic facility should not refuse to care for a patient, even if the facility thought that the patient's refusal was suicidal. That issue is not relevant to the care being offered. The facility should continue to offer care, and by their solicitude for the patient, seek to persuade the person to change his or her view. Discharging suicidal patients would only surrender them to circumstances that may do less to try to persuade them to accept care that is in their best interests.

I am concerned about some gaps in the discussion:

1. What is the obligation to continue to offer life-prolonging treatment that is considered reasonable care, when a person has refused that treatment with the intention of bringing about death, and what is the obligation to continue to care for the patient in other ways?
2. Should a Catholic facility provide palliative care, including pain relief to relieve distressing symptoms caused by dehydration or starvation, when the symptoms could be relieved by hydration or feeding?
3. Should a Catholic facility persist with the course of respecting the person's wishes when secondary psychiatric illnesses develop as a result of dehydration or starvation that preclude the patient from functioning competently or from being able to change her mind?
4. If the person is incompetent, and the decision not to deliver hydration or nutrition is made by a legal representative, such as a guardian, or person with an enduring power of attorney for medical treatment, or the senior available next of kin, or there is a legally valid and binding advanced directive or living will refusing nutrition and hydration, should the hospital comply with that request?
5. Does the fact that, in most jurisdictions, the law permits reasonable force to be used to prevent suicide, change anything with respect to the refusal of medical treatment that is not overly burdensome, or refusal to eat, because the person wishes to die?

2.4.3 The Obligation to Provide Care

I am of the view that a Catholic facility should do its best to persuade a person, who is refusing nutrition and hydration in order to die, to change his or her mind. It should call upon the best of its counselling and other services to that end, but the facility should not act coercively and neither should it withdraw other forms of care. It has a duty of care to do the best by the patient and that includes seeking to persuade them of the right course of action. It would not be in the person's best interests were the facility to withdraw from care so that the he or she is forced to be cared for elsewhere, and perhaps somewhere that does not seek to persuade the person to accept feeding.

There are some who seem concerned that a course of action in which a hospital continues to care for persons refusing nutrition and hydration could be seen as cooperating with the evil of suicide by omission. In my view, a hospital and its staff are restrained by a person's refusal. The permission of the patient, explicitly or implicitly, directly or indirectly, is required for intervention other than emergency treatment. This view is supported by Pope Pius XII:

> The rights and duties of the doctor are correlative to those of the patient. The doctor, in fact, has no separate or independent right where the patient is concerned. In general he can take action only if the patient explicitly or implicitly, directly or indirectly gives him permission.[16]

The issue for the facility and the treating team is different from the issue for the patient. When the treating team is confronted by a patient's suicidal project, the problem is whether they have a right or a duty to provide treatment to prevent suicide. That issue is complicated by the fact that such intervention could only be taken against the patient's wishes. The treatment, then, is not straightforward. It is difficult to feed someone against their wishes as any parent of a two

---

16 Pope Pius XII, "Address to 1st International Congress on Histopathology of the Nervous System" 14/9/52.

year old would testify. One way of achieving this would be by restraining the patient, administering an anaesthetic and performing surgery to install a percutaneous endoscopic gastrostomy tube (PEG tube). Thereafter the PEG tube would have to be protected by physically restraining the patient from pulling it out, or otherwise preventing its use. I would expect that such a course would at least be regarded as "overly burdensome" and beyond the duty of care, even if not itself considered unethical on the grounds suggested by the teaching of Pope Pius XII.

Force-feeding the patient is thus excluded. The obligation to give witness to the truth is met by the concerted efforts of the staff to persuade the patient against suicide, and by their continuing to provide other care.

2.4.4 Palliative Care

A complication in the care of patients who refuse nutrition and hydration arises in regard to the moral acceptability of providing palliation to overcome the discomfort associated with dehydration or starvation, neither of which are comfortable ways to die.

Dehydration is the more problematic because it is associated with severe muscle cramps and severe headaches. Later, as the dehydration causes renal failure, other symptoms associated with the concentration of urea and other blood toxins and imbalance of electrolytes can make the patient feel nauseated, and suffer itch and other pain. There are also cognitive effects that are discussed in the next section.

Starvation is uncomfortable initially as the patient feels hunger, but once that hurdle is crossed at around two weeks, a state of lethargy[17] can prevail as organ shrinkage gradually occurs. The danger of major organ failure develops, including the possibility of liver or cardiac failure, and that may involve pain and distress.

---

17 Dlugoborski, Waclaw, and Piper, Franciszek (eds), *Auschwitz, 1940–1945: Central Issues in the History of the Camp* Five Vols. Oświęcim: Auschwitz-Birkenau State Museum.; Mattson MP 2005; "Energy intake, meal frequency, and health: a neurobiological perspective", *Annual Review of Nutrition*, Volume 25, pp. 237–60.

Palliative care in circumstances in which the patient's discomfort would best be managed by hydration and or nutrition might be seen as cooperation in a suicidal project. It could be argued that the patient's suicidal project is being facilitated by the palliation of the distressing symptoms that follow from being deprived of proper hydration and nutrition.

Faced with an isolated case, it may well be legitimate to provide palliative care on the basis that the pain is genuine and the patient is in need of pain relief and the alternative of administering food and water is not available to the staff because it is refused. It is the issue of public scandal that makes the matter troubling; however, this is addressed by giving witness to the view that ending one's life in this way is immoral, and by continuing efforts to persuade the patient to accept food and water.

2.4.5 Secondary Psychiatric Illness

Withdrawal of nutrition and hydration over time, leads to secondary mental illness: The effects of severe dehydration include loss of comprehension, confusion and disorientation;[18] the cognitive effects of starvation are difficulty concentrating, apathy and poor judgment. The emotional effects of starvation may be depression, anxiety, irritability, anger, changing moods, psychotic episodes, withdrawing from friends and family, and changes in personality.[19]

The patient will, in either case, pass through a phase before death in which he or she is not capable of making decisions and may be unable to review the decision to withdraw hydration and/or nutrition. At that time, the matter becomes an issue for a represented decision, either involving an advanced directive, or a third party, to make decisions on the patient's behalf. The rights and obligations of a third party, as a matter of morality or of law,

---

18 http://nutrition.suite101.com/article.cfm/the_effects_of_dehydration#ixzz0lE4fAb4z

19 http://www.ehow.com/facts_5526044_physical-side-effects-starvation.html

may be different from those of the competent patient. The status of what may amount to a suicidal advanced directive may also be problematic.

From the perspective of those who are caring for the person and who seek to persuade him or her to accept food and water, the loss of capacity to decide otherwise is problematic. In the Rossiter case, having won the case granting him a right not to receive food and water, Mr Rossiter decided not to exercise that right. That someone might refuse and then later change their mind, especially as the symptoms became difficult, cannot be excluded. Therefore the earlier refusal cannot be considered to be binding once the patient has become incompetent and unable to reverse the decision.

2.4.6 Represented Decisions

The question of mental competence, whether prior to a person's decision to refuse nutrition or as a consequence of such a decision, raises an issue about the rights and obligations of representatives and whether their decisions can be rejected.

In the address referred to above, Pope Pius XII also notes:

> What we say here must be extended to the legal representation of the person incapable of caring for himself and his affairs: children below the age of reason, the feeble-minded and the insane. These legal representatives authorized by private decision [power of attorney] or by public authority [guardianship], have no other rights over the body and life of those they represent than those people would have themselves if they were capable. And they have those rights to the same extent. They cannot, therefore, give the doctor permission to dispose of them outside of those limits.

Morally, the representatives have a moral obligation not to bring about the death of the patient by omission, and an obligation to provide care, though not care that is ineffective or overly burdensome.

As a matter of law, at the time of writing, in Australian jurisdictions, the representatives have obligations to act in the best interests of the patient, and this term has statutory definitions that may vary from State to State. The Victorian Definition is:

> for the purposes of determining whether any special procedure or any medical or dental treatment would be in the best interests of the patient, the following matters must be taken into account:
>
> A. the wishes of the patient, so far as they can be ascertained; and
> B. the wishes of any nearest relative or any other family members of the patient; and
> C. the consequences to the patient if the treatment is not carried out; and
> D. any alternative treatment available; and
> E. the nature and degree of any significant risks associated with the treatment or any alternative treatment; and
> F. whether the treatment to be carried out is only to promote and maintain the health and well-being of the patient; and
> G. any other matters prescribed by the regulations.

The law in relation to representatives is thus different from the rights of the patient. The patient can refuse treatment that is in his or her best interests, but the representative may not. Thus, for instance, a patient could make an altruistic choice, such as to donate a kidney while alive, but someone acting on his or her behalf could not do so. The normal course of action to take, should a representative act against the interests of a patient, is to apply to have their status as representative reviewed by a Court or Tribunal.

The law would thus seem to differ from the teaching of Pius XII, who taught that the representative has the same obligations as the patient. There is ambiguity, however, as to whether a third party who acts outside the moral limits has the same status as a competent patient. In other words, might health professionals be able to override the represented decision of a third party, even though they cannot override the decision of the patient?

In the Australia context, I would advise that representation by third parties that are not in the best interests of the patient should be taken for review to a Court or Tribunal.

This would then raise the prospect that, when dehydration or starvation has reached a point that the patient is no longer considered competent, a decision should be sought from a representative, and challenged by seeking review of representation, if he or she opted for death by omission. The Court or the Tribunal might then decide whether the refusal, as a continuation of the person's view of the matter, would be in the person's best interests. I regard such a step as necessary because, while a person is competent it is always possible that they might change their mind, and that possibility should not be considered to be lost because they have become incompetent. Factors that might influence the person to change their mind while competent, should still have a bearing on the person who represents the person when they become incompetent. For instance, it is not uncommon for people to allow family factors to influence decisions about end of life care. One might prefer that one's death not coincide with a family event such as a wedding or the birth of a child. The decision to refuse treatment by the representative may not be as simple as merely continuing what the patient had previously expressed.

There is a further complication in situations where a patient has documented his or her wish to refuse nutrition or hydration in an advanced directive or living will. In this situation, it is a matter for a Court or Tribunal to determine the status of such a directive. A key issue to be considered is whether the patient's project is suicidal, or whether the representative's project is homicidal (see the discussion below).

One of the issues that the Courts will need to resolve is that an approval of suicidal uses of advanced directives would make it very likely that people with suicidal intentions, including young people, would complete advanced directives refusing any attempt to reverse the consequences of their action. I have seen just such a circumstance in an Accident and Emergency Department. They treated because there was no time to assess the circumstances and validity of the documentation. Their decision was supported by the

Supreme Court of Victoria. I have written and published on this matter elsewhere.[20]

In practice, the health professionals attending an attempted suicide will take emergency action to reverse the attempt. The issue about advance directives and refusal normally arises later when emergency treatment has stabilised the situation and there is time to consider the issues. However, if an advanced directive exists, it is not unlikely that the patient's representative might be standing by the bedside refusing all emergency treatment while waving the documents endorsing that decision.

Legal advice would be needed in the presence of an advanced directive, as the statutory status of advanced directives differs across the different jurisdictions.

Within Australia, in Queensland advanced directives cannot be used to refuse food and water[21] and in most States they do not have a statutory status. In Victoria, the refusal of medical treatment is limited to a current condition, and a lapse into incompetence would be a different condition. In approving the legislation, the Parliament explicitly rejected giving a statutory status to an advanced directive. That was the purpose of limiting the refusal to a current condition. Under the Victorian legislation, decisions on behalf of incompetent people depend on the appointment of someone to make decisions on their behalf.

Some have argued that advanced directives have common law validity, but that has been as yet untried in Australian jurisdictions.

I would advise that when faced with an advanced directive refusing food and water, hospitals or other care facilities should seek legal advice as to whether its staff may rely on the law that allows them to intervene, forcibly if necessary, when there is a reasonable suspicion of suicide. This is discussed in the following sections.

---

20 Nicholas Tonti-Filippini "Some Refusals of Medical Treatment which Changed the Law of Victoria", *Medical Journal of Australia*, Vol 157, August 17 1992.
21 *Powers of Attorney Act 1998* (Qld) and the *Guardianship and Administration Act 2000* (Qld).

2.4.7 Use of Reasonable Force to Prevent Suicide

In Australian jurisdictions, the criminal law makes provision for reasonable force to be applied to prevent suicide when there are reasonable grounds for believing that the patient is attempting suicide. In the circumstances of imminent death, it is unlikely that a refusal of treatment, including nutrition and hydration, would be regarded as suicidal, but refusal of nutrition and hydration, by an otherwise well person, would be likely to be seen as suicidal, and may justify intervention to prevent suicide.

For instance, the Victorian *Medical Treatment Act* (1988) explicitly mentions that the Act does not affect the operation of section 6B of the *Crimes Act*, with respect to aiding and abetting suicide, and section 463B of the *Crimes Act* which provides that every person is justified in using such force as may reasonably be necessary to prevent the commission of suicide or of any act which he believes on reasonable grounds would, if committed, amount to suicide. It was clearly the intention of the Victorian Parliament not to allow the law to be used to facilitate suicide. The other States have similar provisions allowing the prevention of suicide and to prohibit aiding and abetting suicide. (See discussion of this issue in the chapter on the Patient's Right to Say No.)

The legal issue of using reasonable force to prevent suicide is relevant to circumstances in which a patient's refusal of what is considered ordinary or non-burdensome care would result in death. It has a particular application when the patient reaches a stage of weakness and inability to make decisions, when care could be provided without difficulty and the hospital would seem to have a duty of care to do so.

2.4.8 Conclusion

It is my preference that a Catholic facility make clear its willingness to care for people who refuse to receive nutrition and hydration, while continuing to seek to persuade them to accept nutrition and hydration. Even if the patient's intent is suicidal, it is my view that this response offers the best chance of saving life. Provided that every reasonable effort is made to offer nutrition and hydration, then I would not consider such care to be cooperation in suicide.

There should always be a presumption in favour of nutrition and hydration. A Catholic facility should always be on the side of supporting the patient to accept it, even if it is not obligatory. At the same time, it should be made clear that if the means are overly burdensome, nutrition and hydration are not obligatory and a person has the moral right to refuse them.

Where a secondary psychiatric illness develops and where there is representation by way of a third party or advanced directive not to accept food and water, then legal or tribunal advice should be obtained as to whether this is in the best interests of the patient. Likewise, advice should be taken in regard to the relevance of the law that allows for the use of reasonable force to prevent suicide.

If the law upholds a represented decision to refuse food and water, then the facility and the professional staff have an obligation not to cause scandal. They should make it clear that they do not endorse the refusal of treatment which aims to cause death by discontinuing care that could readily be provided without causing undue burden. They ought also to continue to offer nutrition and hydration and to seek to persuade the patient or the representative to accept that care. But their obligation would not extend to demanding the discharge of the patient or to the forceful administration of food and water. To do the former would be a lost opportunity, and to do the latter would be unlawful. The latter would therefore risk the capacity of the facility and the staff to continue to provide care and potential loss of employment.

2.5 Euthanasia

Euthanasia is usually qualified as voluntary, non-voluntary or involuntary, and active or passive.

Voluntary euthanasia describes a decision, made freely by a person, to have his or her life ended by another in order to end suffering.

Non-voluntary euthanasia happens when the person is incapable and the decision is made by others to have his or her life ended in order to end his or her suffering.

Involuntary euthanasia is a decision made, against the person's known wishes, by others in order to end suffering by ending his or her life.

People often make a distinction between *active* euthanasia, in which a fatal intervention such as a drug overdose is given in order to end the suffering by ending the life, and *passive* euthanasia, in which life-prolonging treatment is deliberately withdrawn in order to end the suffering by ending the person's life.

The Catholic Church, however, makes no such distinction and has declared that euthanasia in the strict sense is understood to be an action or omission which, of itself, and[22] by intention causes death, with the purpose of eliminating all suffering. Euthanasia's terms of reference, therefore, are to be found in the intention of the will and in the methods used. Pope John Paul II asserts that euthanasia is a grave violation of the law of God, since it is the deliberate and morally unacceptable killing of a human person.[23]

In other words deliberately ending someone's life by a fatal treatment or fatally withdrawing treatment is considered immoral.

The Church does, however, make a distinction between passive euthanasia or killing by omission and withdrawing or withholding treatment that is futile (that is, ineffective) or overly burdensome:

> Euthanasia must be distinguished from the decision to forego so-called "aggressive medical treatment," in other words, medical procedures which no longer correspond to the real situation of

---

22 Note that in earlier versions of this definition of euthanasia a disjunct "or" was used – "of itself **or** by intention". It is not clear why this was changed in the later statement. I have discussed this issue at length in Tonti-Filippini, Nicholas "*Vel* and *Ut*: A Puzzle in the definition of Euthanasia", *New Blackfriars,* Vol 86 No. 1006, November 2005.

23 Pope John Paul II, *Evangelium Vitae* Vatican 25 March 1995, n. 65 Accessible from: http://www.vatican.va/holy_father/john_paul_ii/encyclicals/documents/hf_jp-ii_enc_25031995_evangelium-vitae_en.html.

the patient, either because they are by now disproportionate to any expected results or because they impose an excessive burden on the patient and his family. In such situations, when death is clearly imminent and inevitable, one can in conscience "refuse forms of treatment that would only secure a precarious and burdensome prolongation of life, so long as the normal care due to the sick person in similar cases is not interrupted." Certainly there is a moral obligation to care for oneself and to allow oneself to be cared for, but this duty must take account of concrete circumstances. It needs to be determined whether the means of treatment available are objectively proportionate to the prospects for improvement. To forego extraordinary or disproportionate means is not the equivalent of suicide or euthanasia; it rather expresses acceptance of the human condition in the face of death.[24]

Simply expressed, therefore, euthanasia may be defined as deliberately bringing about death by active intervention (e.g. overdose) or by neglect of reasonable care (e.g. withholding non-burdensome treatments (such as nutrition and hydration/antibiotics) in order to end suffering.

The following are common arguments (in italics) used to support legalizing euthanasia[25] and some responses to them.

1. *If society recognises the autonomy of individuals by granting them the right to pursue their views about the good life, and create their own lives, then the logical consequence is to allow people to decide their own death.*

   Respect for autonomy can mean simply respecting a person's choices whatever he or she decides, or it can mean respecting a person because he or she has autonomy or free will. The distinction becomes apparent when a choice such as suicide or taking

---

24 Ibid.
25 These were drawn from a variety of pro-euthanasia sites including: http://www.exitinternational.net/; http://www.saves.asn.au/; http://www.dwdv.org.au/Legislative Charter.html.

drugs prevents a person from making choices or diminishes his or her capacity to do so. Is it respecting autonomy if we support a decision that a person makes to end any opportunity for autonomy in the future? One of the fathers of modern libertarianism, the philosopher Immanuel Kant, thought that suicide was wrong because it involved treating oneself as an object or a means to end. He himself endured a long illness with cancer.

2. *Since one of the main aims of medicine is to relieve suffering, it is a medical duty to relieve the intractable suffering of a patient by assisting him or her to die.*

Virtually all the national medical organisations in English speaking countries have rejected the idea of physician-assisted suicide because it conflicts with the role of a doctor in seeking to maintain health and life. They say that giving doctors the authority to end the lives of their patients would undermine trust and confidence in them, and for the chronically ill and frail elderly, it would increase the fear that they are a burden to others, and they could feel that they should take the option of euthanasia, if it were available. Suffering is complex and often requires a multidisciplinary effort to manage it. The possibility of euthanasia would shift the focus away from those efforts, and palliative care would lose its political momentum if euthanasia were an option. Suffering cannot always be totally overcome, but there are always ways to assist a person who is suffering and central to those efforts is the notion that the person is valued and important. Euthanasia implies that there are some lives that are not worth living and therefore some people who are valueless. Euthanasia thus contradicts the goals of palliative medicine.

3. *The sacredness of human life is a religious belief. The law should not enforce religious beliefs. When there is a division in society between the right to die with dignity and religious claims about the sanctity of human life, legislation that prohibits assistance to die for a person who is so ill that he or she can no longer enjoy life, and wants to die, is undemocratic and unjust.*

The inviolability of human life is not exclusively a religious notion. International human rights law recognises the right to life as the only right to be declared inherent.[26] A right is inherent when it belongs to the person as a permanent characteristic of that person. Democracy means government for the people and by the people, and it respects the worth of every member of the human family. To declare that some citizens do not have the same protection under the law would be undemocratic. Legalising euthanasia would involve declaring that respect for the lives of those who are chronically ill is not inherent but depends on whether they maintain the will to live. That, in itself, creates a pressure on them to relieve others of the burden of their lives.

4. *There is a difference between the physical or biological life and the biographical life – that which gives it meaning; for example, dreams, aspirations, achievements. If that is lost, then there is no person because the person's distinctive value is lost. The sanctity of life no longer applies to a human who has lost all the characteristics that make him or her a person.*

People who are in an unresponsive state remain as members of the human family, they remain someone's son or daughter, mother or father, sister or brother. Respect for their lives remains inherent because it is based not on their contribution but on who they are. Biographical life is not separable from biological life – dualism is mistaken. We are not two people, but one person who experiences life as a body. It is as that unity that we are respected as members of the human family. When people live in an unresponsive state, the fact of the matter is that we do not know what is occurring. Unresponsiveness does not mean that a person cannot be conscious or can never be conscious again. Consciousness is not observable, but a state that we infer from a person's behaviour. We cannot infer

---

26 United Nations, *International Covenant on Civil and Political Rights* Clause 6. Accessed from: http://www2.ohchr.org/english/law/ccpr.htm.

unconsciousness from unresponsiveness.[27] We simply have to give the benefit of the doubt and do what we reasonably can to sustain people in this state and to keep them comfortable. This was discussed in volume one in relation to the Australian Health Ethics Committee *Ethical Guidelines for the Care of People in Post Coma Unresponsiveness (Vegative State) or a Minimally Responsive State.*[28]

5. *Human life is sacred. The value of human life should not be degraded by reducing the quality of life for the sake of extending the quantity of life. When a person has no quality of life, then he or she should be able to choose to die.*

People are entitled to refuse medical treatment that they consider to be overly burdensome. No-one is obliged to do everything possible to sustain life. The ethical issue concerns recognising the nature of the human condition and the reality that death is a part of life. When death is inevitable, then it is important not to overload the person with futile or overly burdensome efforts to prolong life, but to accept the dying process. However it is impossible to assess the quality of a person's life. We can talk about the quality of objects for which we have some use or purpose, but to talk of the quality of a person's life, is to consider the person an object, not a person.

6. *Withdrawal of life-saving treatment is permissible under the law. The effect of such a decision is the same as administering a fatal treatment. The two acts are morally indistinguishable. In fact, administering a fatal treatment would often be more humane than starving someone to death, letting him or her die of dehydration, or drown in sputum through not treating pneumonia. The law should be consistent.*

---

27 National Health and medical Research Council, *Ethical Guidelines for the Care of People in Post Coma Unresponsive or a Minimally Responsive State* Australian Government 2008, p. 4 Accessed from: http://www.nhmrc.gov.au/_files_nhmrc/file/publications/synopses/e81.pdf.

28 Ibid.

As was argued earlier, and in volume one, it is not appropriate to starve or dehydrate someone to death if it can reasonably be avoided. It is always wrong to deliberately bring about someone's death. However, there can be circumstances in which the available treatments become overly burdensome and the person, or someone acting on an incompetent person's behalf, has a right to refuse treatment that he or she considers to be overly burdensome. The law recognises a right to refuse treatment, though it also upholds a right to intervene with reasonable force where there is a reasonable belief that a person intends suicide. The right to refuse treatment is therefore not an absolute right. The distinction turns on whether there is a reasonable belief that there is suicidal ideation. Refusing treatment because it is overly burdensome does not indicate suicidal ideation. Refusing food and water, when it can be delivered without significant difficulty, or burden, would indicate suicidal ideation, and may provide grounds for intervention that was not overly burdensome. However in my experience with prisoners hunger-striking, it would be overly burdensome to attempt to feed and hydrate someone against their will.

7. *The arguments against euthanasia are mainly slippery-slope arguments. Euthanasia legislation can be drafted so that the practice is safe.*

It is often argued that if voluntary euthanasia is allowed then that would soon be widened to include non-voluntary euthanasia of those who are suffering but unable to speak for themselves. The arguments are supported by history, especially the contemporary experience of the Netherlands where the category of those for whom euthanasia is allowed has gradually widened from those adults who are suffering intractably and choose death for themselves to those who are incompetent, and then more widely to include those who are mentally ill and to children, and more recently there is lobbying to extend it to those who are simply elderly and wish to die because they are "tired of life". These responses provide the first mention of a "slippery slope" argument in this volume; we have seen that euthanasia is not wrong merely in terms of what it might lead to, it is wrong because of what it does, in the here and now, in declaring that some people do not have the same protection of the law and that respect for their lives depends on them having a continuing will to live. The will to live is likely to be affected by the presence of the option of euthanasia and the likelihood that people may then feel they that should rid others, such as their family, of the burden of their continued existence. Euthanasia implies that some lives are not worth living and thus undermines the goals of palliative care, which holds all people to be valuable and worth assisting. The chronically ill and the frail elderly need our love and our support to live as fully and as meaningfully as possible during the dying process.

2.6 Physician-Assisted Suicide

There has been a recent trend towards legislation to provide for physician-assisted suicide. From a medical perspective the main reasons for opposing such legislation are:

1. Medically "assisted dying" in any form undermines the trust in patient-doctor relationships.
2. It changes the role of physician from someone who heals and cares to someone who takes life, thereby corrupting the fundamental ethos of medicine and radically altering the nature and context of aged and palliative care.
3. It puts at risk the fate and wellbeing of our most vulnerable and dependent patients, who already carry with them a deep concern of their burden on others.
4. It endangers the respect and value that society places on human life, especially for those who are sick, disabled and vulnerable, and those who are near the end of life.

Virtually all national medical organizations throughout the English-speaking world, including the World Medical Association, the Australian Medical Association, the British Medical Association, the Canadian Medical Association, the American Medical Association and the New Zealand Medical Association, are unanimous and unequivocal in their rejection of the concept and practice of euthanasia and physician-assisted suicide/dying as unethical and contrary to the ethos of medical care.

Their positions reflect a long tradition of wisdom and ethics in healthcare which recognises the dangers that any form of "medically-assisted dying" may pose to the vulnerable, the sick and the dying, as well as the risks of undermining the nature of the patient-doctor relationship and of corrupting the integrity of medicine.

Such opposition is in keeping with the deeply held values and ideals that have informed the practice of healthcare in the West for almost 2,500 years dating back to the time of Hippocrates.

The Hippocratic Oath, which includes the first recorded statement of opposition to the concept of euthanasia as a practice that is contrary and alien to the fundamental ethics of medicine, states: "I will not give a lethal drug to anyone even if I am asked, nor will I advise such a plan."[29] This simple statement has set the standard for the ethical care of the sick and the dying for millennia; it continues to inform the almost universally accepted ethical norms of caring for the sick and dying, and is reflected in the policy statements of almost every national medical association.

For example, the World Medical Association, which represents 82 countries, in its "Statement on Physician Assisted Suicide" in May 2005 succinctly reiterated its position: "Physician-assisted suicide, like euthanasia, is unethical and must be condemned by the medical profession. Where the assistance of the physician is intentionally and deliberately directed at enabling an individual to end his or her own life, the physician acts unethically."[30]

---

29 http://www.nlm.nih.gov/hmd/greek/greek_oath.html Accessed 1/6/2008.
30 http://www.wma.net/e/policy/p13.htm.

Likewise the Australian Medical Association's "Position Statement on the Role of the Medical Practitioner in End of Life Care," which was published in 2007, stated the association's opposition to euthanasia and physician-assisted suicide and declared that "medical practitioners should not be involved in interventions that have as their primary intention the ending of a person's life."[31]

The British Medical Association (BMA) in June 2006 voted with an overwhelmingly majority against the legalisation of euthanasia and physician-assisted suicide in the United Kingdom, confirming its previously long-held opposition. This occurred soon after the rejection of Lord Joel Joffe's "Assisted Dying Bill" by the House of Lords by a large majority in May 2006.

The subsequent policy statement of the British Medical Association declared that it:

i. believes that the ongoing improvement in palliative care allows patients to die with dignity;
ii. insists that physician assisted suicide should not be made legal in the UK;
iii. insists that voluntary euthanasia should not be made legal in the UK.

In the statement, the BMA stated clearly its opposition to "all forms of assisted dying," remarking that "the primary goal of medicine is still seen as promoting welfare, protecting the vulnerable and giving all patients as good a quality of life as is possible." It rejected the possibility that this "should include deliberately shortening their lives" even "when terminally ill patients request that or when an individual's suffering cannot be fully alleviated." It also confirmed: "Assisting patients to die prematurely is not part of the moral ethos or the primary goal of medicine and, if allowed, could impact detrimentally on how doctors relate to their own role and to their patients." It specifically rejected the

---

31 http://www.ama.com.au/web.nsf/doc/WEEN-76S8CY.

'absolute autonomy' argument for euthanasia stating "that there are limits to what patients can choose if their choice will inevitably impact on other people."[32]

This BMA policy statement recognizes the intrinsic risks and dangers that the "concept of 'assisted dying' poses to the vulnerable and the sick, with whom a doctor's prime responsibilities lie... If assisted dying were an option, there would be pressure for all seriously ill people to consider it even if they would not otherwise entertain such an idea... Health professionals explaining options for the management of terminal illness would have to include assisted dying. Patients might feel obliged to choose it for the wrong reasons, such as if they were worried about being a burden or concerned about the financial implications of a long terminal illness." It recognised that it would seriously "risk undermining patients' ability to trust their doctors and the health care system. In particular, it could generate immense anxiety for vulnerable, elderly, disabled or very ill patients."

The New Zealand Medical Association in its policy statement "Euthanasia and Doctor-Assisted Suicide", published in July 2005, states that "The NZMA is opposed to both the concept and practice of euthanasia and doctor assisted suicide. Euthanasia, that is the act of deliberately ending the life of a patient, even at the patient's request or at the request of close relatives, is unethical. Doctor-assisted suicide, like euthanasia, is unethical." Importantly, it also states that "the NZMA position is not dependent on euthanasia and doctor-assisted suicide remaining unlawful. Even if they were to become legal, or decriminalised, the NZMA would continue to regard them as unethical."[33]

The Canadian Medical Association states that it "does not support euthanasia or assisted suicide [and] urges its members to uphold the principles of palliative care."[34]

---

32 http://www.bma.org.uk/ap.nsf/Content/assisteddying?OpenDocument&Highlight=2,euthanasia.
33 http://www.nzma.org.nz/news/policies/euthanasia.html.
34 http://policybase.cma.ca/dbtw-wpd/Policypdf/PD07-01.pdf.

Finally, despite the unique circumstances of the state of Oregon in the United States, the American Medical Association continues unequivocally to reject all forms of euthanasia. Its policy statement declares that: "Euthanasia is fundamentally incompatible with the physician's role as healer, would be difficult or impossible to control, and would pose serious societal risks" and "would ultimately cause more harm than good." The statement also recognizes the very real risks posed by euthanasia to incompetent and vulnerable patients and recommends that "instead of engaging in euthanasia, physicians must aggressively respond to the needs of patients at the end of life. Patients should not be abandoned once it is determined that cure is impossible."

The ethos and integrity of medicine is rooted in the reverence for all human life and the basic respect for the intrinsic dignity of all members of the human family. This does not allow for a discriminatory approach to the treatment or care of any patient, especially those who are in most need of such help and support. To do otherwise, to mark out some people for "assisted dying," is to devalue the humanity of the sick and dying and to practise the abandonment of the most vulnerable. As a society we should never confuse "caring" with "killing," nor should we make some members of our society eligible to be considered "beyond caring for."

Rather than enabling choice, legalising physician-assisted suicide would increase the likelihood that the chronically ill and the frail elderly would feel that they were a burden, and should take the option, made available, to end their own misery and that of those around them. Their lives would hang on the tenuous thread of their own desire to continue.

Rather than considering legalising physician-assisted suicide, the political emphasis should be on ensuring adequate services for the chronically ill and frail elderly. Palliative care is particularly important. Its main function is to assist people to live more fully during the dying process by relieving distress and, in a multi-disciplinary way, ensuring that their social and emotional needs are met also. Facilitating their suicide would both decrease the political pressure to ensure that there are adequate services available for the chronically ill and frail elderly, and decrease the sense of worth of these vulnerable people.

2.7 The Fragility of Living a Burdensome Life[35]

2.7.1 Introduction

In the previous two chapters, the focus was on the debate over proposals for legalising euthanasia and patient assisted suicide. In fact, several jurisdictions have already done so, and there are other developments that pose a risk to those of us who fit the criteria. Further, the campaigns for change in themselves are not without effect on us. Living a burdensome life has already become much harder and more fragile.

In Western countries, there is a relentless effort by advocates of euthanasia to effect change to the law, either directly by proposing changes to the criminal law statutes, or by seeking regulatory guidelines in relation to the enforcement of the criminal law so that "mercy-killing" in defined circumstances is not prosecuted. The latter was the route taken in the Netherlands, with guidelines issued by the Royal Medical Society that became established practice, and only relatively recently supported in statute law. The initial medical guidelines permitted assisted suicide for the terminally ill, if:

- The patient's decision is voluntary, well considered and persistent
- There is unbearable pain without hope of improvement.
- The decision should be made by more than one doctor, and the doctor and patient should agree that euthanasia is the only reasonable option.

---

35 This chapter began as a letter to Australian Senators and the South Australian Premier. It has been republished several times including in Tonti-Filippini, Nicholas, "Euthanasia and the Fragility of Living a Burdensome Life", *Nova et Vetera*, English Edition, Vol. 9, No. 3 (2011): 561-565.

However, in 30 years from this restricted beginning, the Netherlands moved:

- from assisted suicide to euthanasia,
- from euthanasia of people who are terminally ill to euthanasia of those who are chronically ill,
- from euthanasia for physical illness to euthanasia for mental illness,
- from euthanasia for mental illness to euthanasia for psychological distress or mental suffering, and
- from voluntary euthanasia to non-voluntary euthanasia or as the Dutch prefer to call it "termination of the patient without explicit request."[36]

More recent there has been advocacy for permitting euthanasia in the Netherlands for those who are merely "tired of life".

A similar process has developed in the UK, with the Crown Prosecution Service issuing guidelines for assisted suicide, citing six public interest factors for not prosecuting including:

- The victim had reached a voluntary, clear, settled and informed decision to commit suicide.
- The suspect was wholly motivated by compassion.
- The actions of the suspect, although sufficient to come within the definition of the crime, were of only minor encouragement or assistance.
- The suspect had sought to dissuade the victim from taking the course of action which resulted in his or her suicide.
- The actions of the suspect may be characterised as reluctant encouragement or assistance in the face of a determined wish on the part of the victim to commit suicide.

---

36 Hermina Dykxhoorn Accessed 24/12/10 from http://www.euthanasia.com/netherlands.html.

Care of the Sick and the Dying 109

- The suspect reported the victim's suicide to the police and fully assisted them in their enquiries into the circumstances of the suicide or the attempt and his or her part in providing encouragement or assistance.[37]

Belgium (*Act on Euthanasia* May 2002[38]) and the US State of Oregon followed the more direct route of immediate statute change. On October 27, 1997, Oregon enacted the *Death with Dignity Act* which allows terminally-ill Oregonians to end their lives through the voluntary self-administration of lethal medications, expressly prescribed by a physician for that purpose.[39]

In Switzerland, an old law has been interpreted to allow assisted suicide. Article 115 of the Swiss penal code considers assisting suicide a crime, if and only if, the motive is selfish. It thus condones assisting suicide for altruistic reasons. In most cases the permissibility of altruistic assisted suicide cannot be overridden by a duty to save life. Article 115 does not require the involvement of a physician nor that the patient be terminally ill. It only requires that the motive be unselfish.[40]

In seemingly all Western jurisdictions, there is recognition of the right to refuse medical treatment and the latter, through withdrawal of life prolonging treatment such as withdrawing provision of nutrition and hydration and non-treatment of infection, is also a way in which euthanasia or assisted suicide may be achieved.

Lack of ethical and legal clarity, in this respect, has provided a relative easy route to achieve non-voluntary euthanasia. Sedation and demand feeding, for those who are not competent, (including

---

37 Crown Prosecution Service, "DPP publishes assisted suicide policy" 25/02/2010 Accessed 26/12/10 http://www.cps.gov.uk/news/press_releases/109_10/.
38 Accessed 26/12/10 from http://www.kuleuven.be/cbmer/viewpic.php?LAN=E&TABLE=DOCS&ID=23.
39 http://www.oregon.gov/DHS/ph/pas/ accessed 26/12/10.
40 Hurst, Samia A, Mauron, Alex "Assisted suicide and euthanasia in Switzerland: allowing a role for non-physicians", *BMJ* 2003; 326 : 271, 1 February 2003.

newborn infants with abnormalities and whose parents accept that option), have provided a means of achieving non-voluntary euthanasia. In the case of infants, the death can thus be achieved for a child who does not suffer from a terminal illness, but is merely disabled and not wanted by the parents.

There are thus diverse ways in which the prohibition of mercy-killing in most western jurisdictions may be set aside, and the protected status of some ill or disabled people may be altered to allow them to be killed or assisted to die. The existence of a person who lives a burdensome life has therefore become very fragile in our society.

Apart from lawful killing, there are also some indications that a small proportion of health professionals are willing to take the law into their own hands even in circumstances in which it is unlawful.[41] Where it is lawful, there are also indications that doctors will practice euthanasia outside of the legal requirements.[42]

2.7.2 A Personal Perspective

I write this article as a person whose protected status would be likely to be affected were the jurisdiction where I reside to change the law to permit euthanasia. I have accounted elsewhere for my illnesses (See Chapter Five in this volume and also the Preface to *About Bioethics, Volume One: Philosophical and Theological Approaches*). Suffice to say that I have had a chronic degenerative illness for more than thirty years, renal failure and ischaemic heart disease, and, being immune compromised, several near fatal episodes of illness.

I cannot speak for all people who suffer from illness and disability, but think I can speak more credibly about suffering, illness and

---

41 Baume P, O'Malley E. Euthanasia: attitudes and practices of medical practitioners. *Med J Aust* 1994; 161: 137–145; Wadell, Charles. Clarnette, Roger M. Smith, Michael. Oldham, Lynn. Kellehear, Allan. "Treatment decision-making at the end of life: a survey of Australian doctors' attitudes towards patients' wishes and euthanasia", *MJA* 165 (540).

42 Van Der Maas PJ, Van Delden JJ, Pijnenborg L, Looman CW. "Euthanasia and other medical decisions concerning the end of life" *Lancet*. 1991 Sep 14; 338(8768):669-74.

disability than those people who advocate for euthanasia. Often the latter present an ideological view of suffering and disability that does not reflect the reality. Facing illness and disability takes courage, and we do not need euthanasia advocates to tell us that we are so lacking dignity, and have such a poor quality of life, that our lives are not worth living.

Professionally, I have been involved with issues to do with the care of the sick and terminally ill for many years, having been Australia's first hospital ethicist, thirty years ago, at St Vincent's Hospital, Melbourne, where I was also Director of Bioethics for a period of eight years. Since then, I have been a consultant ethicist in private practice and have taught ethics in the medical faculties of the University of Melbourne and Monash University, before taking my current position at the John Paul II Institute. The Institute is associated with the Lateran University in Rome and is a registered Higher Education Provider in Australian offering accredited specialist graduate courses in Bioethics and in Theological Studies in Marriage and Family.

Also relevant, is that recently I had the experience of chairing a National Health and Medical Research Council (NHMRC) Working Committee conducting a public enquiry and preparing guidelines for the care of people in an unresponsive state, or a minimally responsive state. How we care for people who are so disabled is closely related to this topic of euthanasia. The strength of submissions from people who care daily for Australia's most dependant and needy individuals was overwhelming and I highly recommend that you read the public submissions on the NHMRC's web-site or at least read the NHMRC *Ethical Guidelines for the Care of People in an Unresponsive State or a Minimally Responsive State (2008)*. Importantly, the guidelines provide a careful analysis of the way in which care decisions may be made so as to preserve respect for the dignity and worth of people who are so profoundly disabled, and to provide care for the families and others who care for people with PCU or MRS.

I have also had a long-term association with a home hospice service that serves the eastern area of Melbourne. I would like to record my own view that it would not benefit seriously ill people, particularly those who are terminally ill and suffering intractably, if the Commonwealth *Euthanasia Laws Act* 1997, which prohibits euthanasia in Australia's territories, was rescinded. The current legal situation while not perfect, does provide a measure of protection against the terminally ill being regarded as a burden. As a chronically ill person, I know well what it is to feel that one is a burden to others, to both family and community, how isolating illness and disability can be, and how difficult it is to maintain hope in the circumstances of illness, disability and severe pain, especially chronic pain.

For several years, until I objected, I received from my health insurer a letter that tells me how much it costs the fund to maintain my health care. I dreaded receiving that letter and the psychological reasoning that would seem to have motivated it. Each year I was reminded how much of a burden I am to my community. The fear of being a burden is a major risk to the survival of those who are chronically ill. If euthanasia were lawful, that sense of burden would be greatly increased for there would be even greater moral pressure to relinquish one's hold on a burdensome life. Seriously ill people do not need euthanasia. We need better provision of palliative care services aimed at managing symptoms and maximising function, especially as we approach death. Rather than help to die, the cause of dignity would be more greatly helped, if more was done to help people live more fully with the dying process.

2.7.3 Further Problems with Euthanasia Legislation

The proposal to make provision for a terminally ill person, who is suffering, to request, and a doctor to provide, assistance to die, makes it less likely that adequate efforts will be made to make better provision for palliative care services. Legalised euthanasia would give those responsible for funding and providing palliative care a political "out", in that respect.

In many jurisdictions, too little is done to make adequate palliative care available to those who need it:

- Current entry requirements for palliative care usually exclude people with chronic pain and is often limited to people who are in the last stage of cancer[43] with a prognosis of less than eight weeks;
- Government pharmaceutical subsidies, where they exist, for the more effective forms of pain relief are often restricted to cancer patients;
- People living outside major cities often have little access to palliative care facilities.
- Few doctors are adequately trained to provide palliative care.
- Such palliative care services as exist are chronically underfunded and struggle to provide the complex range of services that are needed to assist a person to live with pain and disability.
- Most pain clinics are over subscribed and have long waiting lists. For people who are left suffering, such waiting is unconscionable.

Medical research in this area indicates that the desire for euthanasia is not confined to physical or psychosocial concerns relating to advanced disease, but "…incorporates hidden existential yearnings for connectedness, care and respect, understood within the context of the patients' lived experience. Euthanasia requests cannot be taken at face value, but require in-depth exploration of their covert meaning, in order to ensure that the patients' needs are being addressed adequately".[44] In most jurisdictions, what is needed is often not available or not available in time. It is distressing to note that in the US State of Oregon in 2009, none of the patients who were lawfully

---

43 There are efforts to broaden the diagnostic criteria to include the terminal phase of other illnesses, and some services already admit non-cancer patients.

44 Yvonne, Yi, Wood, Mak and Glyn, Elwyn "Voices of the terminally ill: uncovering the meaning of desire for euthanasia" *Palliative Medicine*, Vol. 19, No. 4, 343–350 (2005).

killed at their own request were referred for formal psychiatric or psychological evaluation. It is also distressing to note that it is reported that two thirds of people lawfully killed under euthanasia laws, in those jurisdictions that permit it, are women.[45]

If euthanasia or assisted suicide were to become a legitimate option with a determined structure, such as was the case in the Australian Northern Territory for a brief period, and is the situation in Switzerland, Belgium, the Netherlands and Oregon, then life for the chronically seriously ill would become contingent upon maintaining a desire to continue in the face of being classified as a burden to others. Essentially such legislation or guidelines involve setting up a category for people whose lives may be deliberately ended. Their protected status as a member of their communities depends on a contingency. Passage of such legislation would imply that our community considers that our continued survival depends on us not succumbing to the effects of pain and suffering, depends on us not losing hope.

In the Netherlands, Attorney General T.M. Schalken found that Dutch society has already undergone transformation in relation to attitudes to the sick and the elderly. As a consequence, some groups reportedly live in fear and uncertainty. The Dutch Patients' Association stated in 1985 that "in recent months the fear of euthanasia among people has considerably increased."[46]

Chronically ill people need the unequivocal protection of their lives. We need protection and encouragement from our community; we do not need this form of discrimination. Far from protecting the dignity of those who are seriously ill and suffering, a euthanasia law would undermine dignity by undermining our sense of individual worth as a person, no matter our suffering and disability.

It should be noted that of the seven deaths that happened under the terms of the Rights of the Terminally Act in the Northern

---

45 Wolf Susan M., "Gender, Feminism, and Death: Physician-Assisted Suicide and Euthanasia," in Susan M. Woolf (ed.), *Feminism and Bioethics*, Oxford University Press, 1996, pp 282-317.

46 "Suicide on Prescription," *Sunday Observer* (London, England), 30th April 1989, p. 22.

Territory of Australia that permitted euthanasia, four did not actually meet the criteria.[47] The legislation was manifestly unsafe and I would argue that legislation that permits euthanasia could never be made safe for those of us who have serious chronic illnesses, because the essence of such legislation is to make respect for our lives contingent upon the strength of our will to survive. Such legislation depends on each of us, who has a serious illness and is suffering, not losing hope. If euthanasia is lawful then the question about whether our lives are overly burdensome will be in not only our minds, but the minds of those health professionals and those family members on whose support and encouragement we depend. The mere existence of the option will affect attitudes to our care, and hence our own willingness to continue.

That desire to live is often tenuous in the face of suffering and in the face of the burden our illnesses impose on others, our families and the wider community. Politicians would gain nothing worthwhile for us by supporting the legalisation of deliberately ending the lives of those who request death. Such requests warrant a response in solidarity from our community, a response that seeks to give us more support and better care, rather than termination of both life and care.

Often these proposals contain safeguards such as:

- Requirements for two doctors, including a specialist, to examine the person making the request.
- Demanding a psychiatrist be consulted if either doctor believes the person is not of sound mind or acting under "undue influence".
- Creating some kind of bureaucracy to register euthanasia and even having powers to intervene if a relevant medical practitioner believes a request for euthanasia should not be granted.

---

47 Kissane, David W, Street, Annette, Nitschke, Philip, "Seven deaths in Darwin: case studies under the Rights of the Terminally Ill Act, Northern Territory, Australia", *The Lancet,* 1998 Vol 352: 1097-1102.

- Strict restrictions on witnesses, jail terms for misleading statements, and a ban on for-profit centres and the promotion of voluntary euthanasia by insurance companies

However there are usually many practical problems with such legislation including:

- The legislation is likely to have a very wide scope, it affects not just those who are imminently dying. The definition of "terminal illness" includes people who may be months or years away from their illness causing death. As a person whose life depends on extraordinary care, including haemodialysis for four x four hour sessions each week, on that basis alone, I fit the description. I also have severe angina throughout those sessions, caused by the haemodynamics of the treatment and my own compromised coronary flows, and I have many other episodes of pain throughout the day, including waking at night in pain. Whether that is a profound level of pain and/or distress depends on the support that I receive from those close to me, as much as it depends on my own will. That euthanasia is not offered to me is important to that response. People who are ill and disabled need that support and encouragement and the knowledge that those around them value them.
- The legislation is often ideologically driven and seldom if ever has been generated by a broad-based enquiry that takes into account the interests of all citizens, and especially those with chronic or terminal illness. The approach is almost always narrow, and does not address the provision of adequate care and support for those in need. The motives for the enquiries appear to be more a matter of ideology than a genuine attempt to respond to the range of matters that affect us. The focus is almost always on the issue of killing, not on bettering the circumstances of people who are chronically ill. If only the effort and the resources expended on euthanasia enquiries could have been devoted to exploring how care of those in need of palliative care could be improved.

If those who support euthanasia were genuine in their advocacy, they would focus broadly on what is needed to better the circumstances of those whose interests they claim to represent, rather than on ways to making killing them lawful.
- The legislation would expect the doctors involved to prescribe a drug, not for legitimate purposes that define the medical vocation, such as the care of the patient or the treatment of illness, but to intentionally and actively intervene to end the life of the patient. In that respect, such legislation is not supported by the major medical associations. For instance, the Australian Medical Association's policy on euthanasia is to "strongly oppose any bill to legalize physician-assisted suicide or euthanasia, as these practices are fundamentally inconsistent with the physician's role as healer."[48]
- The legislation is not supported by organizations and institutions directly involved in aged care, the care of the dying or the care of those with chronic illness. Those involved in the day to day care are generally not in favour of being given the capacity to end the lives of those they care for.
- The legislation would make protection of the lives of those who are chronically ill dependant on the strength of their will to continue. The fear of being a burden is a major risk to the survival of those who are chronically ill. If euthanasia were lawful, that sense of burden would be greatly increased for there would be even greater moral pressure to relinquish one's hold on a burdensome life and to remove that burden from the lives of others.
- The legislation usually uses a notion of "unbearable pain", or words to that effect. A major part of pain experience, and our capacity to tolerate it, is what is sometimes called "existential pain". Pain of an existential nature arises usually from loneliness and a lack of sense of self worth. The option of euthanasia provides an "out" for families and carers, and the fact that the

---

48 http://www.ama-assn.org/apps/pf_new/pf_online accessed 15/5/08.

option exists would be likely to make someone who had a burdensome illness feel even less valued and increase the likelihood that they would choose death over dying alone, or being a burden to others. Serious illness and dying are times when a person needs the support of others so that others can share empathy with that person.[49] The possibility of opting instead for a fatal prescription, would cast a shadow over those relationships and would be likely to undermine the person's wish to be wanted and valued. Imagine the different feeling there would be in the household of a sick person if the bathroom cabinet was known to contain the prescribed lethal dose, awaiting that moment when the sick person, or perhaps someone else, decides that the moment has arrived.

- Pain and suffering are complex, involving physical, psychological, emotional and spiritual elements. Palliative care seeks to address the needs of those who are suffering in a multi-disciplinary way that reflects the many elements involved.[50] Crucial to good palliative care is the support of the patients socially, emotionally and spiritually. It is not simply a matter of relieving physical pain. For those who continue to live with a burdensome illness, the option of euthanasia would undermine one of the essential elements of good pain relief, the notion that the person is supported, loved and wanted.
- In places, such as the United Kingdom, for instance, which have adopted very liberal policies on other social policies, such as reproductive technology, gay unions and abortion, the Parliaments have strongly opposed euthanasia because euthanasia cannot be made safe for people who are seriously ill, and thus vulnerable. It is worth noting that jurisdictions, such as the

---

49 Yvonne, Yi, Wood, Mak, and Glyn Elwyn "Voices of the terminally ill: uncovering the meaning of desire for euthanasia", *Palliative Medicine*, Vol. 19, No. 4, 343-350 (2005).

50 Hudson, Peter, Kristjanson, Linda J, Ashby, Michael, Kelly, Brian, Schofield, Penelope, Hudson, Rosalie, Aranda, Sanchia, O'Connor, Margaret, Street, Annette.(2006) "A systematic review of the desire for hastened death in patients with advanced disease and the evidence base of clinical guidelines" *Palliative Medicine* 20, 693-71.

Netherlands and Belgium, that legalised euthanasia, lacked the availability of the kind of palliative care services that had developed in the UK.
- Euthanasia law cannot be made safe. The Northern Territory of Australia briefly legalised euthanasia, for a brief period before it was overturned by a Commonwealth law. As discussed above, several of those for whom the legislation was implemented did not in fact meet the criteria of the Act despite the safeguards.[51] This is reflected also in the Dutch experience where much larger numbers than were expected have been subject to the law, raising human rights concerns.
- Euthanasia is contrary to the international human rights instruments. When the Human Rights Committee of the United Nations considered a euthanasia law enacted in the Netherlands to codify what had become euthanasia practice, the Committee said that, where a State party seeks to relax legal protection with respect to an act deliberately intended to put an end to human life, the Committee believes that the International Covenant on Civil and Political Rights obliges it to apply the most rigorous scrutiny, to determine whether the State party's obligations to ensure the right to life are being complied with (articles 2 and 6 of the Covenant). The Committee expressed the concerns that the new Act (in the Netherlands) contains a number of conditions under which the physician is not punishable when he or she terminates the life of a person, inter alia at the "voluntary and well-considered request" of the patient in a situation of "unbearable suffering", offering "no prospect of improvement", and "no other reasonable solution". The Committee also expressed concern lest such a system may fail to detect and prevent situations where undue pressure could lead to these criteria being

---

51 Kissane, David W, Street, Annette, Nitschke, Philip, "Seven deaths in Darwin: case studies under the Rights of the Terminally Ill Act, Northern Territory, Australia", *The Lancet*, 1998 Vol 352: 1097–1102. Note that one of the authors, Nitschke, was a major proponent of the Northern Territory legislation.

circumvented. The Committee was also concerned that, with the passage of time, such a practice may lead to routinization and insensitivity to the strict application of the requirements, in a way not anticipated. The Committee learnt with unease that, under the present legal system, more than 2,000 cases of euthanasia and assisted suicide (or a combination of both) were reported to the Netherlands' review committee in the year 2000, and that the review committee came to a negative assessment only in three cases. The large numbers involved raise doubts whether the present system is only being used in extreme cases in which all the substantive conditions are scrupulously maintained.[52]

---

52 http://www.unhchr.ch/tbs/doc.nsf/0/dbab71d01e02db11c1256a950041d732?OpenDocument&Highlight=0,euthanasia, accessed 26/5/08.

3. Representation and Disability

3.1 Best Interests Decisions vs. Substituted Judgement

3.1.1 Introduction

In 2010, by publishing a Consultation Paper,[1] the Victorian Law Reform Commission invited discussion on matters to do with representation of people who have a disability and need someone to represent them in medical and other decision-making. A crucial issue was that the Commission proposed change to the law, from what was described as respecting the *best interests* of the person, under an accepted practical formula that included the person's wishes and values, to a *substituted judgement* in which the decision would represent exclusively what were understood to have been the wishes of the patient, as determined by the representative.

The issue is complex, especially in relation to medical treatment decisions, because it involves a tension between individualism and communitarianism in public policy, that has particular moment in relation to people with disabilities who may be dependant on others to implement their decisions, and who may be more than usually reliant on the family or other community in which they live, and the community in which they may work. Second, the distinction also involves competing notions of what it means to respect a person's dignity. Some regard the meaning of dignity as being exhausted by the concept of autonomy. Others understand it as also including a notion of the worth of the person and their development and flourishing. This debate has particular moment in the representation of people whose disability affects their capacity to make reasoned choices, such as

---

[1] http://www.lawreform.vic.gov.au/wps/wcm/connect/justlib/Law+Reform/Home/Current+Projects/Guardianship/LAWREFORM+-+Guardianship+-+Consultation+Paper+Summary.

those with cognitive impairment. A richer notion of dignity is needed in that instance than mere autonomy.

The Commission's view in favour of substituted judgement represents a broader contemporary trend in relation to representation of people with physical disabilities who may need to be represented because of their vulnerability to others, as well as people whose decision-making may be temporarily or permanently impaired, such as people with developmental disabilities, dementia, cognitive disabilities resulting from trauma or disease, or people with mental illness. It seemed worth discussing some major matters raised by the Commission because they reflect a broader trend toward a doctrinaire individualism and away from communitarianism, despite the dependence, often, of represented people on communitarian attitudes and assistance.

In adopting substituted judgement, the Commission also proposed a uniform approach to all the different areas of representation, making representation of medical treatment decisions no different from representation for property, financial or accommodation matters. However, there are quite different aspects in relation to medical treatment decisions, and decisions with respect to people who suffer from a mental illness or an intellectual incapacity, on the one hand, and other decisions that may need to be made for a person, such as accommodation, property or financial decisions. Substituted judgement might be fine for financial decisions, but is a problem for health decisions.

3.1.2 Medical Treatment Decisions are Different

In relation to medical treatment, in the Australian State of Victoria, the *Medical Treatment Act* 1988, the *Mental Health Act* 1986, the *Disability Act* 2006 and the *Guardianship and Administration Act* 1986 are designed to deal with quite different needs for representation and different relationships and contexts, than is needed for decisions involving only accommodation, property and financial matters. Legislation with respect to health and mental health involves very significant responsibilities for the State with respect to individual health, life and liberty.

In principle, there is no reason why the several statutes that deal with representation of people could not be in the one piece of legislation, but it is important that the different needs and contexts are reflected in the ways in which representation is appointed, and the principles that guide representatives. For instance, unlike other decisions, the power to make a medical treatment decision is relevant to the law in relation to aiding and abetting suicide and the law of homicide.[2] What may be permissible for a competent person to decide, may not be permissible for an agent: suicide is not an offence but aiding and abetting suicide is. That difference also applies in relation to non-therapeutic medical procedures. For instance, a competent individual may be free to make an altruistic decision to be a living organ donor, but, as the National Health and Medical Research Council has concluded, a representative ought not to have the power to make such a decision on the person's behalf.[3] Altruism cannot be exercised on someone else's behalf, because altruism involves personal sacrifice. When a person decides for another, it is not altruism.

If there were to be one piece of legislation, the legislation would need to define and separate the different areas of need for representation and the requirements for each. Representation should not be a single mode or method for all areas, but needs to provide for separate decisions for the different needs. The person who might make medical treatment decisions will often be a different person, with very different responsibilities from the person one might appoint to make financial decisions, and the State has very different responsibilities to

---

2 *The Medical Treatment Act* 1988 states:

This Act does not –
a. affect the operation of section 6B(2) or 463B of the Crimes Act 1958; or
b. limit the operation of any other law.

3 National Health and Medical Research Council, *Organ and Tissue Donation by Living Donors – Guidelines for Ethical Practice for Health Professionals*, Australian Government Printer 2007 http://www.nhmrc.gov.au/_files_nhmrc/publications/attachments/e71.pdf.

ensure accountability and that the necessary requirements are met. Handing over decisions about one's health, life and liberty to someone else is quite different from handing over management of a share portfolio. In making decisions about representation, people typically choose persons for these roles based on their specific competencies in each area.

Arguably the capacity to make medical treatment decisions and decisions about the freedom of a person with mental illness or intellectual incapacity should be separated from other types of decisions by representatives, because of the very different responsibilities of the State to protect life, which is the only right in the international human rights instruments to be considered inherent as well as being inalienable.[4]

3.1.3 Dignity and Representation

The Commission proposed a new purpose for the legislation:

> *The purpose of this Act is to protect and promote the dignity and human rights of people with impaired decision-making capacity. To this end, the Act establishes mechanisms to support and assist people to participate in decisions that affect their lives, realise their rights and protect their inherent dignity.*

The concept of dignity is a vexed issue in this context. The second sentence refers only to the participation of people in their decisions. In fact the function of guardianship law is to authorise and guide someone else to make decisions on another's behalf when they are not, or are no longer, able to make their own decisions. It is a laudable goal to try to have the represented person participate in those decisions and to realise their rights and protect their dignity. However, for the most part, the legislation needs to be directed to those others who are authorised to make those decisions, in order to secure the rights and dignity of someone else, and directed to those

---

[4] *International Covenant on Civil and Political Rights* n. 6 http://www2.ohchr.org/english/law/ccpr.htm.

agencies who monitor and review whether they do, and to health and other professionals who, in seeking to serve the interests of a represented person, are guided by the representative and need the latter's consent.

Given the State's obligation to protect the individual's life, liberty and security, the statement of purpose, especially the first sentence, lacks a great deal of qualification, in relation to the *inalienability and equality* of rights and *inherent* human dignity. These words are used in the international human rights instruments because they have an essential meaning. Referring to the rights of people with impaired capacity is ambiguous and does not make plain that, as members of the human family, they have *equal* rights and those rights cannot be lost, taken or given away – they are *inalienable*. There are no special rights for people with a disability, as the statement seems to imply, they have the same rights as everyone else, and they can never lose them.

The referral to dignity in the first sentence is vague as to its meaning. In the international human rights instruments the term "inherent dignity" means both respect for autonomy and respect for the worth and inviolability of the person. The inclusion of the word "inherent" is intended to imply that they have dignity simply by being a member of the human family and that dignity is retained even if they lack autonomy. Inherent dignity thus includes respect for their worth or inviolability.[5]

Relevant to the issue of autonomy and inviolability is the reality that people can make competent choices that are contrary to their dignity. They can willingly risk harm or damage to themselves, risk their lives, or opt to be treated in undignified ways by requesting risky cosmetic surgery for non-medical reasons, taking addictive, mind-altering substances, selling themselves into prostitution, or working in unsafe workplaces. The State might permit some such activities

---

5 Tonti-Filippini, N. (2000). Human dignity: autonomy, sacredness and the international human rights instruments. PhD thesis, Department of Philosophy, The University of Melbourne. http://dtl.unimelb.edu.au/R/6GNFATVP71QDUMI26CFDU2D VNH23RQ1RCQ9NQBX2CQ7DYGK3LJ-00951?func=dbin-jump-full&object_ id=66021&local_base=GEN01&pds_handle=GUEST.

because of the harm done by prohibiting individuals from self harm, but the same consideration might not apply to an exploitative or harmful decision on behalf of a person with a disability. A competent person might choose to be a boxer or to be a prostitute, but the State would need to act if a representative allowed an incompetent person to be beaten up in the ring or engage in prostitution. The State has an obligation to protect people who are made vulnerable by their incapacity to make decisions for themselves.

Finally, the purpose only refers to people with impaired decision-making capacity. There is a difference between autonomy, the capacity to make one's own decisions, and autarchy, the capacity to live independently of the assistance of others. The current legislation[6] recognises the hard fact that sometimes representation is needed for a person who has a disability, not because he or she cannot make decisions, but because he or she is so physically dependent on someone else for day to day living, that freedom to make decisions is affected, and he or she is vulnerable to being exploited or neglected.

3.1.4 Autonomy, Autarchy and Dependence

A person may be fully competent to make their own decisions and therefore is autonomous, but physically disabled and therefore dependent on others. Thus they may be autonomous, but lack autarchy. Even with full capacity to make decisions, if I cannot cook, shop or go to the bank, then my choices as to what I have to eat, am entertained by or what I do with my money, may, in large part, be determined by someone else and the extent and goodwill of their cooperation with me. That often involves compromises, because it involves dependence on relationships. In the real world of living with a disability, and often needing to depend on the goodwill of others, life may not be so free. Relationships are complex and protecting

---

6 The *Guardianship and Administration Board Act* 1986 serves any one who has a disability and needs representation: "The purpose of this Act is to enable persons with a disability to have a guardian or administrator appointed when they need a guardian or administrator."

human dignity does need to take into account a person's context and family circumstances, perhaps dealing with the family unit, in order to best protect the rights and dignity of a person with a disability, because the goodwill and cooperation of those others is necessary to the person's interests. The individualism[7] that underlies the Commission's approach to dignity, breaks down in the circumstances of dependence on others through disability.

It is puzzling that the purpose of the document, referred to above, does not address those whose cooperation is vital, if the rights and dignity of people who need representation are to be protected, and does not address the responsibility of the State to monitor representation to protect rights and dignity, particularly the life, health, freedom and security of people who depend on others. This is a major goal of legislation of this kind. The purpose of the document might therefore be amended to the effect:

> *The purpose of this Act is to protect and promote the inherent dignity and equal and inalienable human rights of people with impaired decision-making capacity and, those who through disability are vulnerable, because they depend on others. To this end, the Act establishes mechanisms to*
>
> - *support and assist people to participate in decisions that affect their lives as far as their disability permits,*
> - *appoint and guide their representatives, and*
> - *revise representation when it fails to protect them, especially their life, health, freedom and security.*

---

7 Individualism is usually contrasted with communitarianism, which emphasizes the importance of community in the functioning of political life, in the analysis and evaluation of political institutions, and in understanding human identity and well-being. According to communitarians, liberalism relies on a conception of the individual that is unrealistically atomistic and abstract; it also places too much importance on individual values such as freedom and autonomy. The Church takes a view that is communitarian in that it upholds the dignity of the human as linked to the vocation to be in communion with others expressed in the command to love God and neighbour. See for instance: Taylor, Charles *The Ethics of Authenticity* Harvard University Press Cambridge, Massachusetts and London, England 1992.

Alternatively, the Commission might have applied the purposes stated in the *Convention on the Rights of People with Disabilities:*[8]

> The purpose of the present Convention is to promote, protect and ensure the full and equal enjoyment of all human rights and fundamental freedoms by all persons with disabilities, and to promote respect for their inherent dignity.
>
> Persons with disabilities include those who have long-term physical, mental, intellectual or sensory impairments which in interaction with various barriers may hinder their full and effective participation in society on an equal basis with others.

The purpose of the Convention at least picks up the broad nature of impairments and treats disability as something that happens as an interaction with the social and physical environment, and treats dignity as inherent and not exclusively determined by possessing autonomy. However, this latter statement still lacks the specificity of the issues to do with representation, and the need to guide and review their role.

3.1.5 Representation is Needed when Relationships Breakdown

There is an essential inconsistency between the individualism expressed by the Commission and the *Convention on the Rights of Persons with Disabilities*. The preamble to the Convention recognises that disability is an evolving concept, and that disability results from the interaction between persons with impairments and attitudinal and environmental barriers that hinders their full and effective participation in society on an equal basis with others.

The crucial notion that is recognised within the field of disability is that the major barriers to participation are not the impairment suffered by the individual, but the attitudes of those around them, and the failure to provide accessible environments. To remove those barriers to inclusion requires the cooperation and goodwill of others.

---

8 http://www.un.org/disabilities/default.asp?id=150.

The individualism of the language of "rights and empowerment" of the Commission misses the point, altogether, that representation is done by someone else and the legislation needs to address the broader context of the best interests of the person as a member of a family or community.

The need for representation is not for the normal circumstance when people of goodwill serve the needs of a person who has a disability, respectful of that person's dignity and capacity to make their own decisions. The need for representation occurs when there is a danger of neglect or exploitation because of the person's vulnerability, and dependence on others. That may be because of a lack of goodwill, but it may also reflect a lack of resources available to the person with the disability, and/or those who care for them, and those who represent them.

3.1.6 Rights are Based on Needs rather than Autonomy

The comprehensive list of human rights in the international instruments were included because they are necessary for the development and flourishing of members of the human family and thus essential for dignity.[9] Rights are based on recognised basic human needs. That development and flourishing happens in community, and the needs are met alongside the needs of others. The meeting of needs is most often dependant on the actions of others and on their recognizing and enacting responsibilities, whether that be individuals, communities, corporations or governments.

---

9 The preambles of both International Covenant on Civil and Political Rights and on Economic, Social and Cultural Rights state:

> Considering that, in accordance with the principles proclaimed in the Charter of the United Nations, recognition of the inherent dignity and of the equal and inalienable rights of all members of the human family is the foundation of freedom, justice and peace in the world,
> Recognizing that these rights derive from the inherent dignity of the human person, that, in accordance with the Universal Declaration of Human Rights, the ideal of free human beings enjoying civil and political freedom and freedom from fear and want can only be achieved if conditions are created whereby everyone may enjoy his civil and political rights, as well as his economic, social and cultural rights...

The *Convention on the Rights of People with Disabilities*, in its principles, refers to "full and effective participation and inclusion in society" and "respect for difference and acceptance of persons with disabilities as part of human diversity and humanity", alongside "respect for inherent dignity, individual autonomy including the freedom to make one's own choices, and independence of persons".

The language of rights and empowerment only make sense when it acknowledges that rights are a relationship between the right holder, the right and those who are in duty bound. The typical use of a two term relation – the rightholder and the object of the right, such as, for instance, a right to healthcare, lacks meaning and enforceability, because no-one is duty-bound by it, unless it is assumed that Government signatories are so bound by the right. However many rights depend not only on government, and that is certainly the case for a person with a disability, who is reliant on his or her family or community context. The principles need to address both parties: the person with a disability, and those others in their community who provide essential assistance, representation and protection.

3.1.7 Participation in Representation

It is important to recognise the right of people with disabilities to participate in decisions affecting them, as far as is possible and practicable. In that respect there is a need to acknowledge the need for flexibility in representations of people whose capacity to make decisions may fluctuate, and may be relative to the type of decision to be made. Rather than simply classifying people as in need of representation or not in need, the forms of representations available do need to take into account these variations in need. A person experiencing dementia, for instance, may have quite different capacities at different times of the day depending on tiredness and depending on the effects of medications for dementia or for concurrent conditions. Second, he or she may need assistance to make complex decisions, but be able to make decisions that were less demanding. He or she may well retain a capacity to express long held values that should guide a decision, but need assistance to apply those values to a novel situation. At a general level there is often a need for a continuum of representation that takes into account the variability of need for it.

In this, the proposed move away from the best interests principle that informs the current law toward adopting so-called "substituted judgement" is highly problematic. The move involves the Commission adopting a subjective notion of dignity based on upholding autonomy, rather than the worth and inviolability of all members of the human family. The Commission holds that the decision of the decision maker "should be the decisions that the decision-maker believes the person would have made if they were able to do so". This would be a dramatic change to the laws, making vulnerable people much more available for neglect and exploitation by providing the sole criterion that the neglect or exploitation could be said to have been something that the represented person would have chosen.

The State has a *parens patria* obligation to ensure protection of the best interests of people who are unable to make their own decisions, and that has particular application in relation to matters that affect their dignity and especially danger to their life. As discussed earlier, the criminal law in most Western jurisdictions has no offence for attempted suicide, but it does prohibit aiding and abetting suicide and does provide for the use of reasonable force to prevent suicide, where there exists a reasonable belief that suicide may be attempted. The Victorian *Medical Treatment Act* 1988 is carefully nuanced[10] in these respects to prevent its provisions being misused to override the criminal law or to remove the liability of those who have a duty of care for a patient. If the principle espoused by the Commission were adopted in the law then there would be a conflict with the criminal law. It could, in effect, prevent the prevention and treatment of suicide where the wishes of the would-be suicide were known.

---

10 *The Medical Treatment Act* 1988 section 4(3) states:

    This Act does not –
    a. affect the operation of section 6B(2) or 463B of the Crimes Act 1958; or
    b. limit the operation of any other law.

In the international human rights instruments, the inherent human dignity of every member of the human family is described as the basis of equal and inalienable rights. Dignity therefore cannot be lost by disability. However, as discussed, the Commission shows a tendency to interpret "dignity" subjectively in terms of autonomy alone rather than in terms also inclusive of the worth and inviolability of the person. In the instruments, the worth and inviolability of persons is recognised in the provisions relating to the right to life, liberty and security of person[11], trafficking in drugs[12] or in women,[13] slavery and unsafe work practices,[14] just to name a few rights that people might choose to violate, for these practices violate human dignity even if the person would have chosen them.

There have been recent trends to facilitate sexual intimacy involving persons who suffer from such cognitive impairment that they cannot make the complex decisions involved in forming a sexual relationship, by engaging sex workers or designating staff willing to oblige in that way, with the approval of a representative, despite the possibility that such "services" might be considered technically to be rape or at least a criminal sexual assault.[15] Someone else's consent, other than the victim, has never been a defence to a charge of rape or sexual assault. These circumstances highlight the need for a balanced best interests judgement, rather than a substituted judgement, which transfers all authority to the decision-maker. Currently the tribunal can review representation that fails to take into

---

11 United Nations International Covenant on Civil and Politica Rights, n. 6.

12 United Nations *Convention against Illicit Traffic in Narcotic Drugs and Psychotropic Substances* http://www.unodc.org/unodc/en/treaties/illicit-trafficking.html.

13 *Protocol to prevent suppress, and punish trafficking in persons, especially women and children, supplementing the United Nations Convention against Transnational Organised Crime* http://www.uncjin.org/Documents/Conventions/dcahistoryl_documents_2/convention_%20traff_eng.pdf.

14 *International Covenant on Economic, Social and Cultural Rights* Art 6,7 and 8 http://www2.ohchr.org/english/law/cescr.htm.

15 Murray, Suellen and Powell, Anastasia, *Sexual assault and adults with a disability: Enabling recognition, disclosure and a just response,* Published by the Australian Institute of Family Studies. Issues no. 9 2008.

account other matters in the person's best interests than the narrow criterion of whether he or she is estimated by the representative to have expressed a wish for a certain outcome or process. The deliberate sexualisation of people who are cognitively impaired raises very serious issues about what is in their interests that go far beyond what their wishes may be. Recently the Family Planning Association of New South Wales released a new Policy and Procedural Guide for disability service providers. Launched by former Justice Michael Kirby I April 2011, the guide aims to assist people with disabilities to access sex workers. He observed that, "Touching Base [the name of the guide] is trying to develop a liaison, a contact, a conversation between sex workers and people with disabilities" and to "deny sexual expression to human beings, cuts them off from that aspect of their personalities and of their happiness and you have a lot of very frustrated and very unhappy people."[16] It is an odd but nonetheless not uncommon notion in contemporary society that one has to be sexual active to be healthy. This is an issue that raises profound questions about whether sexualisation of people with cognitive disabilities could be considered to be in their interests, the impact that it has on their relationship with other staff who are not available for sexual services, and the consequences of heightened sexual awareness and demand from people with cognitive disabilities, who may find it difficult to recognise the social limits of their behaviour. There is a need for decisions to reflect their best interests and not just their expressed wishes.

3.1.8 Representation in Mental Health Decisions

The Victorian *Mental Health Act* 1986 necessarily deals with decisions by health professionals to compulsorily treat people against their wishes, clearly overriding their autonomy in their best interests and the interests sometimes of others, and, because it gives individuals this power, it contains a different set of principles and standards for

---

16 http://www.fpnsw.org.au/127580_3.html.

representation, accountability and review. It would be most unfortunate if a desire for uniformity and simplicity were to lose these very important principles and standards in mental health care.

In these respects there is deep concern about the suggestion that substituted decision-making should displace decisions in the best interests for people who are represented in medical and mental health decisions. The current balance in the best interests principle ensures that best interest decisions include the values and wishes of the person who is represented. Anything that decreases the capacity to review the nature of representation in these matters would be to the disadvantage of those who need representation and whose life and health may be at risk.

3.1.9 Best Interests versus Substituted Judgement

As discussed, the Commission wishes to remove best interests as the basis of represented decisions and instead adopt substituted consent. The current laws require represented decisions to be in the best interests of the represented person. The Victorian *Guardianship and Administration Act* 1986 states for the purposes of determining whether any special procedure or any medical or dental treatment would be in the best interests of a patient, the following matters must be taken into account –

  a. the wishes of the patient, so far as they can be ascertained; and
  b. the wishes of any nearest relative or any other family members of the patient; and
  c. the consequences to the patient if the treatment is not carried out; and
  d. any alternative treatment available; and
  e. the nature and degree of any significant risks associated with the treatment or any alternative treatment; and
  f. whether the treatment to be carried out is only to promote and maintain the health and well-being of the patient; and
  g. any other matters prescribed by the regulations.

This, then, is the "best interests principle", and reflects the necessary balance involved in making a decision for someone else. It is a mixture of factors that goes beyond whether the decision would be chosen by the represented person. Importantly, the Act permits a concerned person to seek to have the representation reviewed, on the grounds that the decision might not be in the best interests of the patient, even if he or she had never articulated those concerns.

The current law recognises that representation is more than just about autonomy, and in that way recognises the essentially complex nature of the position that a representative is in. He or she must take into account a mixture of factors that are involved in ensuring that the person receives adequate care including the person's values and wishes but also the relationship to and the goodwill of others, often family members, and the effects of the decision upon the person and those others.

In reality, and as reflected in the current law, a person's representative is guided by the represented person's wishes, but also recognises that he or she is not that person's robot or slave, but has his or her own conscience, and thus a right and obligation to make a practical moral judgement about what is the right course of action to pursue, taking into account, also, the context and relationship to others, and other community obligations. To disregard all of that, and demand instead, that the representative must do as the person would have wanted, lacks perspective and, ultimately, would not protect the interests of the represented person. It would often place the representative in an impossible position of conflict between what is in the best interests of the person, and their past wishes.

There would also be difficulties for health practitioners and their duty of care. It is one thing to have a person, who can speak for him or herself, refuse to comply with reasonable life-saving care. They are unlikely to be forced to accept what is in their best interests because of the harm done by so forcing them. But when a patient is frail, incapable and perhaps unaware, and someone else is making a harmful even homicidal decision on their behalf, the situation is quite different, because no harm is done by intervening in their best interests.

The doctor or nurse's duty of care to take reasonable steps to protect health and life, rests uncomfortably with a refusal by someone else, claiming that they represent his or her wish to die. What may be suicidal, in the one instance, becomes aiding and abetting suicide, and even homicide in the second instance.

The ethical and legal significance of representation of medical treatment decisions is very different from enforcing an unwanted decision on a person who represents him or herself. The practice is for police and others to prevent suicide, and for health professionals to treat suicide attempts, despite representation of refusal.

This move towards substituted consent favours individualism over communitarianism, ignoring the practical reality that people with disabilities often depend on the cooperation and goodwill of others, and the responsibility of the State to secure the life, health and liberty of all its citizens.

The current concept of best interests also provides scope for the very difficult legal and regulatory position a person might be in, because the law does treat decisions made on behalf of someone else differently from decisions that an individual might make for him or herself.

As discussed, the law in relation to suicide, aiding and abetting suicide and preventing suicide is a good example. But it also applies to risk taking. I can take risks on my own account for good reasons such as altruism, or for reasons such as sport, but if someone else is in my care, my obligation to them is different from my obligation to myself. I might still be able to take risks, because that is what they would have wanted, but the burden is on me to show that that is in their best interests. For example, consider a person with swallowing difficulty taking the risk of aspiration for the sheer enjoyment of tasting food, rather than having everything safely delivered safely through a tube. The current best interests' principle allows such a decision, by balancing the wish and the risk.

The substituted consent alternative bases the decision on the wishes of the patient, with no consideration of best interests, nor consideration of those others who are affected by the decision.

When Graham Kinney[17] was brought to St Vincent's Hospital in Melbourne, having suffered an overdose, and accompanied by his wife and brother with a note demanding that he not be treated, the hospital was able to have the representation reviewed and a decision made by the Public Advocate, who replaced his wife as representative. Subsequently, treatment was authorised. That decision was later endorsed by the Victorian Supreme Court. In a substituted consent regime, that capacity to review on the basis of best interests would no longer exist, or, at least, be much more difficult to exercise.

Similarly, the law, at least in practice, might allow a person to possess limited quantities of illicit drugs for private use, but it would regard possession of illicit drugs to give to a person entrusted to one's care very differently.[18]

3.1.10 Conclusion

The move towards substituted consent is not to the advantage of people with disabilities. The most dangerous aspect of it is that it would narrow the scope of the capacity to have representation reviewed.

In aged care facilities, it is not uncommon for a representative to have a conflict of interest. The spouse of a person with dementia may enter into a new relationship, or the children of someone with dementia may want to move on with their inheritance. As the representative, either by appointment or by being the senior available next of kin, they have the power to deny that person ordinary life preserving treatments such as the flu vaccine, antibiotics and even feeding, as well as more invasive treatments. Currently, the facility can challenge such a decision on best interest grounds and seek review of the representation, or threaten to do so, which is often all that

---

17 Tonti-Filippini, Nicholas, "Some Refusals of Medical Treatment which Changed the Law of Victoria", *Medical Journal of Australia*, Vol 157, August 17 1992 pp. 277–9.

18 *Drugs, Poisons and Controlled Substances Act* 1981 sections 70(1) & 71AC).

is needed. Under substituted consent, the representative can claim that the person would not have wanted to live with dementia, and there would be less scope to challenge what is, in effect, a homicidal decision.

3.2 Options for Planning Future Care[19]

Advanced directives are often promoted as a way of ensuring that when you cannot make your own decisions, appropriate decisions are still made. A major problem with such directives is that health professionals may lack information about what you meant, what your state of mind was, and what you understood of the options at the time.

Because illness is seldom predictable, a directive is not likely to be adequately informed. Before a health professional could act on a directive he or she would need to ask:

- Do the present circumstances correspond to the circumstances envisaged at the time when the person recorded his or her wishes?
- Do the treatment and care options available correspond to those about which the patient made his or her statement?
- Do the effects of implementing the patient's wishes correspond to the effects that the patient understood would be their consequence?
- Are there new or changed factors in the present circumstances which the patient may not have taken into account but would have wanted to be considered in the present circumstances?

A better option than issuing a directive is to appoint someone you trust to make decisions for you, and explain to them the values and

---

19 This and the following sub-sections have been adapted from materials I co-authored with Bishop Anthony Fisher OP, Rev Dr Gerald Gleeson and Dr Bernadette Tobin. Our work was published as *A Guide to Future Care Planning* by Catholic Health Australia approved by the Australian Bishops and available as a free download from http://www.cha.org.au/site.php?id=223.

priorities that you would want to be applied. They can then respond to the circumstances as they arise.

Many people prefer to trust in the health professionals, and their family and friends, rather than trying to direct events beforehand. However, in our increasingly secular culture, there may be less and less reason for people with a religious perspective to have that confidence. Further, making end of life decisions can be very difficult for loved ones, and providing them with some indication of your wishes may relieve them of a difficult burden.

3.3 Accepting Death and Dying

As human beings, and especially as Christians, we are called to engage with the reality of the human condition and to take responsibility for the gift of life until death comes. While they are still able to do so, people should accept the inevitability of their own illness and death, and consider the implications for themselves and others.

The Catholic tradition has always emphasised that life is a gift, not a possession. As responsible stewards of this gift, we should seek assistance when sick and generally look after our health and well-being. It is prudent to make known our own preferences for medical treatment, in case we are ever incapacitated and unable to communicate, and it is often a good idea to ensure that there are people who have the authority to make decisions in the event of disability.

For many people, the days leading up to death can acquire a positive, life-giving meaning. Believers accept the unpredictability of the human condition, and, like Jesus at Gethsemane, strive to place their trust in God's will. Accordingly, we should try to accept the unavoidable disability and dependence of our later years, and not expect fully to control the dying process. To some extent, we should leave those entrusted with our care free to respond to the course of illness as it unfolds in the mystery of one's life, rather than attempt to tie their hands with instructions, issued without direct knowledge of those future events.

3.4 Desirability of Future Care Planning

No-one should be compelled to issue instructions about future care. Nevertheless, it is desirable that patients give some guidance about their medical treatment to those who have authority to make such decisions. The best way to do this is by means of someone who is able to speak for the patient when he or she is unable to do so.

People often need time and assistance to reflect on the place of death in their lives, to face and resolve interpersonal differences within families, and to avoid future conflict between family members.

There are different ways in which people can guide their future medical treatment; it is not necessary to leave written instructions. Many people can simply trust their families and their healthcare professionals to know and do what is best for them. In some cultures and ethnic groups, this is the normal way in which healthcare decisions are made.

In all cases, communication between a person, and his or her family, friends and healthcare professionals, is invaluable. It is recommended that patients seek out a personal doctor or nurse practitioner with whom they can develop a good continuing relationship. With the development of trust and understanding, good communication of one's fears, hopes, and desires becomes possible.

Patients need their healthcare professionals to explain the likely course of an illness, the various treatment options available, and their benefits and side-effects.

Health professionals need to hear from their patients about their hopes and goals in life, their relationships with their families and communities, their tolerance of treatment side-effects, their religious commitments, and what will be important to the person as death approaches.

It is best for this communication to occur by means of many conversations over the years with one's family and friends, and with one's doctors and nurses. If conversations about these matters are gradually and gently introduced, then it will be easier to discuss specific and immediate questions when they arise in relation to terminal illness. Fresh opportunities for conversation may occur when there is a change to living circumstances caused by illness or disability.

3.5 How is a Representative Appointed?

Illness and disability may change a person's role in life and status. How each person endures, and the relationships that form through illness and dependency, are an important part of the journey that continues until death. Those relationships continue even when the person's own ability to contribute actively diminishes. For Christians, in becoming more dependent on others, one still has important witness to give to the suffering of Christ.

If a person becomes unable to make decisions for his or her own medical treatment, there are three ways in which someone may be or become that person's representative:

a. The person has appointed someone previously;
b. A court or tribunal appoints someone after the person becomes incompetent;
c. The spouse, carer, other next of kin, or close friend, according to law, may have that authority automatically. The senior available next of kin has that authority in Australian jurisdictions, if no-one else has been appointed by the person or by a court or tribunal.

The representative should be made aware that he or she is likely to have that responsibility, and should be given some guidance about how the role is to be exercised. If a person does not have confidence in those who would automatically have the role of representative, then that person needs to appoint someone of his or her own choosing. In most jurisdictions there are legal processes for doing that.

The advantage of appointing such a person is that he or she is able to respond, on one's behalf, to the changing circumstances in which treatment decisions are needed. While the representative's formal role is to make medical treatment decisions on the patient's behalf, he or she might also have a less formal role in coordinating discussion among the family members, where practicable, and communicating with the treatment team.

A person chosen as a representative should:

a. be able to make good judgements in what may be difficult and painful circumstances;
b. know the person who is represented, and his or her values and wishes;
c. appreciate the person's sense of stewardship in relation to health and life;
d. be likely to be available to fulfil that role should it be needed in the future.

3.6 What to Record?

A person appointing a representative may wish to give some guidance as to how decisions should be made. Some people will simply be happy to discuss what may happen with them, while others may also want to provide their guidance in writing.

There are several ways in which a person's wishes may be recorded:

a. The doctor or nurse may (and normally should) keep his or her own notes of what the person has said, and review them regularly, as they will change as circumstances change.
b. The person may prepare a statement of general principles about what he or she would like done in the future.
c. The person may prepare a specific plan for care in the immediate circumstances of a degenerative illness about which he or she has been well informed. In preparing such a plan, communication with one's doctor is essential because normally only a medical practitioner has the expertise and experience to inform patients of their prognosis and of the treatment options. Guidance from

other healthcare professionals, pastoral carers, ministers of religion or community elders may also be helpful.

In some jurisdictions, advanced directives or advanced care plans have been given a legal status. These are unsatisfactory, because they are likely to be inflexible, and their legal status may prevent doctors and nurses from changing care to suit changes in the circumstances. They may also suggest wording that would refuse care that should be provided or insist on treatment that should not be. It would be better not to use documents that attempt to be *directive*. Rather, one's written wishes should *guide* what happens, while being flexible enough to allow your representative to adjust to new situations on the advice of the doctors and nurses.

3.7 Why Guide the Representative?

A representative will have the role of evaluating medical treatment decisions, if the person represented becomes unable to do so. He or she will need to assess what a particular treatment may achieve and what difficulties it may cause.

By giving guidance to others about future treatment and care, the person represented may relieve the anxiety and burden of decision-making for the representative. Such guidance should respect the representative's responsibility to value and care for the person until death intervenes. A representative takes on the same obligation that each of us has to protect and sustain our own life.

In providing guidance, one can help by considering the possible course of one's illness and indicating one's priorities. We are obliged to use those means of preserving our lives that are effective, not overly burdensome and reasonably available. (Such means are referred to in the Catholic tradition as "ordinary" or "proportionate.") Each person has a moral right to refuse any treatment that is futile, or that he or she judges to be overly burdensome or morally unacceptable, and such refusals must be respected. (Such means are referred to in the Catholic tradition as "extraordinary" or "disproportionate.")

How treatment decisions should be made, by whomever has the authority to make them, is addressed earlier.[20]

A person who has a degenerative disease with a predictable course (e.g. renal failure, advanced ischaemic cardiac disease, metastatic cancer, advanced multiple sclerosis) would normally be informed of the likely progress of the disease, and of the likely benefits and burdens of treatment options, especially in the latter stages. It may help others if the person represented were to think about the circumstances in which he or she would regard some intrusive life-sustaining interventions, such as cardio-pulmonary resuscitation, renal dialysis, or mechanical ventilation, as overly burdensome.

Those without a degenerative illness may nevertheless wish to guide their treatment and care in the foreseeable circumstances of a life-threatening situation (e.g. stroke, heart failure, accident). In such a case, one can give only general guidance about the treatments wanted and the kind of benefits and burdens of treatment that one would judge to be reasonable. A frail, elderly person, for example, might judge that, in the circumstances of an arrest, intubation, cardiac massage and defibrillation (the usual elements of resuscitation) would be overly burdensome. But he or she might want ordinary care to continue in the meantime, including, for instance, antibiotics for infection or assistance with feeding.

The person represented may wish to clarify the burdens on others that he or she would find acceptable, for example, by requesting only the kind of treatment or care that can be provided where he or she lives, without the need for prolonged hospital care.

3.8 More about the Problem of Advanced Directives

I strongly encourage people to appoint someone with an enduring power of attorney for medical treatment (or the equivalent in other jurisdictions) to make decisions in the future, as the Victorian *Medical*

---

20 See for instance section 2.1 in this collection headed "Care of the Dying and Proportionate Means."

Treatment Act provides, and to discuss future health care planning with them. The Australian Catholic Bishops' Conference has supported documents issued by Catholic Health Australia by which people can indicate their wishes, but has not supported issuing binding advanced directives. In a recent submission to the Victorian Law Reform Commission, the Church strongly opposed the issuing of binding instructions (advanced directives or living wills) for several reasons:

a. The Church supports the notion of informed consent and it is unlikely that a directive for future events can be adequately informed. The evidence[21] suggests that because health practitioners have to make a decision at that future time about what the person understood at the time of making the decision, and to interpret what their wishes mean in that new circumstance, advance directives in practice have little effect on decisions. People are better off appointing someone and discussing with them their values and preferences.
b. It is immoral to seek to bind someone else to acting in ways which they may find to be against their conscience. Advance directives are such that they risk violating the right to freedom of conscience, thought and belief.
c. Some of the proposals for advance directives are in effect suicidal, refusing everything, including food and water, that would keep the person alive.

Advanced directives, or living wills, are therefore not appropriate for medical treatment decisions because of their binding nature in circumstances of a lack of relevant information, and because they provide no opportunity for discussion especially when carrying them out may involve ethical difficulties.

---

21 Fagerlin, Angela and Schneider, Carl E., "Enough: The Failure of the Living Will" *The Hasting Centre Report Vole 34* No 2 March-April 2004; Eiser, Arnold R. and Weiss, Matthew D., "The Underachieving Advance Directive: Recommendations for Increasing Advance Directive Completion", *The American Journal of Bioethics*, Vol. 1, Number 4 2001, p. 1-5.

In passing the Victorian *Medical Treatment Act* 1988, the Victorian Parliament rejected the notion of advanced directives. The Act provides for a person to refuse a medical treatment option, but not as an advance directive. The refusal is limited to a current condition only.[22] The purpose of so doing was to prevent the certificates being used as an advanced directive.

Currently, in many jurisdictions the law allows people to provide instructions or wishes when appointing an enduring guardian or an enduring attorney (financial) or its legal equivalent. There are different titles used for the documenting of the power. However in the jurisdictions with which I am familiar, there would appear to be little provided in the practical circumstances for them to enforce such a request. This is not a just a local factor. The evidence internationally,[23] such as in US states that have legislated to enforce advanced directives, indicates that where they exist they play little role in the decisions made. The may get invoked to validate a decision in accordance with them, but otherwise they appear to be largely ignored.

There is a problem with trying to direct future events because of the lack of knowledge about what the future may hold. The reason for appointing someone is to trust in their judgment about what is in

---

22 **Medical Treatment Act 1988 Section 5, Refusal of Treatment Certificate**
  1. If a registered medical practitioner and another person are each satisfied –
     a. that a patient has clearly expressed or indicated a decision –
        i. to refuse medical treatment generally; or
        ii. to refuse medical treatment of a particular kind – for a current condition; and
     b. that the patient's decision is made voluntarily and without inducement or compulsion; and
     c. that the patient has been informed about the nature of his or her condition to an extent which is reasonably sufficient to enable the patient to make a decision about whether or not to refuse medical treatment generally or of a particular kind (as the case requires) for that condition and that the patient has appeared to understand that information; and
     d. that the patient is of sound mind and has attained the age of 18 years – the registered medical practitioner and the other person may together witness a refusal of treatment certificate.

23 See for instance: Fagerlin, Angela and Schneider, Carl E. "Enough: The Failure of the Living Will," *Hastings Center Report* 34, no. 2 (2004): 30–42.

your best interests. This is particularly significant if there are matters of health and life at stake, but seemingly not so personally significant otherwise, though of course financial matters may affect health matters. Where one lives may determine what care is available, and where one lives may be determined by financial decisions.

Suggestions have been made by the Victorian Law Reform Commission[24] that new offences be created for people failing to comply with instructional directives. The issue is one of trust. The purpose of giving a power of attorney is to entrust matters to that person. If there were offences associated with holding a power of attorney, then it would be foolish to be prepared to accept the role, and their function would be undermined and be likely to fall into disuse. I would suggest that the power not be enforceable, but that it be definitely reviewable if there is concern that decisions were being made not in the person's best interests.

Health professionals who encounter a representative who is making decisions not in the patient's best interests, which often happens as discussed earlier, should seek review of the representation in the interests of the represented person.

---

24 Victorian Law Reform Commission, Op. Cit.

4. Ethics and Mental Illness

4.1 What is Mental Illness?

The Australian Department of Health and Ageing advises that mental illness can be defined as a clinically recognisable set of symptoms (relating to mood, thought, or cognition) or behaviour that is associated with distress and interference with functions (that is, impairments leading to activity limitations or participation restrictions).[1] It should be noted that people can have mental illness and still be moderate or even high achievers. It is not uncommon for some high achievers to note that they have bi-polar disorder, for instance. Many people live competently and responsibly, while grappling with severe depression due to mental illness.

The Department's National Community Advisory Group on Mental Health (1994) defined mental health problems as:

> Problems associated with mental illness which if not addressed result in severe disadvantage, continued dependence on mental health treatment and crisis services, and which severely curtail the ability of the individual to live independently in the community to their fullest potential. The problem and the need associated with the problem are understood by reference not only to diagnosis, but also to diagnosis in the context of impact on life circumstances. Problems associated with behavioural and/or personality disorders fall within this definition.[2]

Often severe mental illness is distinguished from other forms of mental illness that many people manage to live with. While there is no agreed definition of these terms, many researchers use the term

---

[1] http://www.health.gov.au/internet/main/publishing.nsf/Content/mental-homeless-toc~mental-homeless-1~mental-homeless-1-3.

[2] Ibid.

"severe mental illness" to apply to psychotic disorders such as schizophrenia and bipolar disorder that are characterised by a loss of sense of reality, auditory or visual hallucinations, thought disorder, and delusions. Other researchers have used more inclusive definitions that include a wider range of mental disorders such as depression, anxiety and substance use disorders. The diversity of definitions used makes it difficult to compare the prevalence rates identified by various studies. It is, however, important to distinguish between *psychosis*, which may include misinterpretation and misapprehension of reality, hallucination, delusion and thought disorder, and *neurosis*, which may include anxiety, phobia, panic, obsessive compulsive disorder, post-trauma syndromes, and psychosomatic disorders.

From an ethical point of view, there is a need to distinguish practically between those who, though affected by mental illness, are still able to comprehend their circumstances and make decisions that are made on the basis of those circumstances, and people who lack that capacity and may need someone to make decisions in their best interests. This distinction, however, is not black and white: competence or the lack of it may be decision-specific. For example, a person who is affected by addiction may lack the capacity to make a competent decision about drug or alcohol use but have no difficulty making decisions about unrelated matters. Mental illness is often episodal, leaving the person to be able to function well enough at other times.

Further, lack of competence to make a decision in given circumstances though mental illness, might not prevent people from giving expression to the values or the relationships that are important to them, or what may be called their "critical interests", those matters of conviction or opinion, whether articulated or not, that are particularly important in an individual's life.[3]

---

[3] National Health and Medical Research Council, *Ethical Guidelines for the Care of People in Post-Coma Unresponsiveness (Vegetative State) or a Minimally Responsive State* Australian Government 2007, p. 48, http://www.nhmrc.gov.au/_files_nhmrc/file/publications/synopses/e81.pdf.

Mental illness needs also to be distinguished from cognitive impairment. In dealing with someone who has a mental illness, one might be dealing with someone who is in fact of very high intelligence. It is sometimes said that the line between being a genius and being mentally ill is very thin.

I have lived closely with mental illness within my own family. Protecting their privacy prevents me from saying more. However, I do wish to record my admiration for anyone who lives with mental illness, the courage and resolve needed so often to complete ordinary tasks at times, and the understanding and strength of perception that often the experience of illness may have given them. I have wondered whether some forms of mental illness are due to an extraordinarily heightened emotional intelligence and awareness, that cuts through the ordinary deceits of life, leaving them aware of extraordinary cognitive dissonance which may challenge their grasp on our ordinarily deceitful reality.

As hospital ethicist, I participated from time to time in medical rounds in psychiatry where difficult ethical cases were discussed, and at other times I reviewed policies from the Department of Psychiatry that had ethical implications. The hospital had a secure ward for prisoners and there was potential for conflict between the hospital policy that prisoners would have the same access to care as anyone else, and the requirements for good order at the prison. I became acutely aware of how sensitive the prison environment is and how difficult it is to maintain order with low staff to prisoner ratios and dependence on prisoner cooperation. The contribution of the environment to mental ill-health is also a matter that was of concern.

4.2 Classifying Mental Illness

Mental illness may have biological and/or psychological origins, and these causative factors may be interrelated. For instance there is some evidence that schizophrenia may be associated with perinatal stress on the mother but also that there may be significant macroscopic changes in the brains of people with the disease and some biochemical changes.[4] One of the diagnostic criteria for borderline personality disorder is that the person reports having been physically or sexually abused as a child.

There are two main English classification systems for mental illness:

- the WHO *International Classifications of Diseases* (ICD -10)
- the American Psychiatric Association (DSM-IV) *Diagnostic and Statistical Manual*

The WHO ICD classification system includes:

a. organic disorders, e.g. stroke, Alzheimer's disease
b. misuse of drugs, e.g. memory loss, addiction
c. schizophrenia and related delusional disorders, e.g. paranoia
d. mood disorders, e.g. depression, bi-polar
e. neurotic disorders, e.g. phobia, panic
f. behavioural syndromes associated with physiological disorders, e.g. anorexia, insomnia
g. disorders of adult personality, e.g. fear of abandonment
h. intellectual disability
i. disorders of psychological development, e.g. autism

4.3 The Significance of a Diagnosis

An important consequence of diagnosis of mental illness may be involuntary treatment. In most jurisdictions, a decision about involuntary treatment is made by a doctor (perhaps requiring corroboration by another or review by a Court or Tribunal) on the grounds that:

a. the person appears to be mentally ill;
b. the person's mental illness requires immediate treatment;

---

4 Arango, Celso and Kahn, René, "Progressive Brain Changes in Schizophrenia" *Schizophr Bull.* 2008 March; Vol 34, No. 2, pp. 310–311.

c. because of the person's mental illness, involuntary treatment of the person is necessary for his or her health or safety (whether to prevent a deterioration in the person's physical or mental condition or otherwise) or for the protection of members of the public;
d. the person has refused or is unable to consent to the necessary treatment for the mental illness;
e. the person cannot receive adequate treatment for the mental illness in a manner less restrictive of his or her freedom of decision and action. A person is mentally ill if he or she has a mental illness, being a medical condition that is characterized by a significant disturbance of thought, mood, perception or memory.

A person is not to be considered to be mentally ill because he or she:

a. expresses or refuses or fails to express a particular political opinion or belief;
b. expresses or refuses or fails to express a particular philosophy;
c. expresses or refuses or fails to express a particular sexual preference or sexual orientation;
d. engages in or refuses or fails to engage in a particular political activity;
e. engages in or refuses or fails to engage in a particular religious activity;
f. engages in sexual promiscuity;
g. engages in immoral conduct;
h. is intellectually disabled;
i. takes drugs or alcohol (without serious temporary or permanent physiological, biochemical or psychological effects);
j. has an antisocial personality;
k. has a particular economic or social status or is a member of a particular cultural or racial group.

It is ethically important to acknowledge clear goals for medical treatment of mental health, including first identifying the problem that is to be treated, which would usually include disturbance of thought, mood, perception or memory that is distressing or causes actions or disability that endanger self or others. Having identified the problem, the goals may include:

a. overcoming distress;
b. overcoming disturbance to ability to make decisions that are reasonably based upon the circumstances;
c. respecting mental, spiritual and bodily integrity.

A diagnosis of mental illness offers explanation of conduct that indicates illness rather than badness, and it thus may provide comfort, assist communication, provide a framework for clinical decisions, help to predict the effects of treatment and selection of treatment, and facilitate research into causes.

There is an important ethical distinction to be made between:

- medicine, which respects the patient, his or her personality and ability to make decisions;
- psychiatric medicine, which recognises deficiencies or pathologies in the patient's personality or ability to make decisions.

Thus in medicine the immediate treatment goal is guided by the patient's own judgments, while the goals of psychiatric medicine may be to alter those judgments.

4.4 Truth telling and Diagnosis of Mental Illness

Truth-telling in medicine is usually important because it assists the patient to make his or her own decisions, and not to tell the truth may be manipulative and coercive, and a failure to respect the patient's dignity and responsibility for his or her health care.

Deception, however, may be a part of caring for someone whose mental illness prevents the making of decisions based on his or her circumstances. Placebos (the use of a "dummy" treatment) can in some instances be an effective form of treatment but this depends on misleading the patient, convincing him or her that the treatment will be effective while administering something that does no harm. Similarly, suppressing information about the side-effects of treatment is known often to reduce the experience of bad side-effects and thus to increase compliance with a helpful treatment, while information about possible effects and side-effects may set up the expectation of such effects, increase their incidence, and therefore increase non-compliance.

This raises issues to do with the sometimes coercive nature of treatments for mental illness. The justifications for coercion include preventing

a. danger to others where psychiatry is used as agent of social protection
b. danger to self where psychiatry is paternalistically protective of the individual on the basis that there are defects in the person's capacity to make adequate decisions informed by his or her circumstances.

4.5 Ranking Psychiatric Treatments by their Capacity to Alter Personality

Primum non nocere – first do no harm – is a central maxim in the practice of medicine. In psychiatry, it is thus important to minimise change to the personality while overcoming the distress or disability caused by the illness. Oddly enough, the effects of treatment are considered by psychiatrists to be the opposite of what a lay person may expect: electro-convulsive therapy is least likely to alter personality, followed by brain surgery, then drug treatment, with psychotherapy the most likely to bring about change in personality.

4.6 The Social Uses of Psychiatry

Mental illness has sometimes been classified wrongly as criminality, in circumstances when, in fact, the illness prevented the person from having sufficient understanding to form the intent to commit crime. Under such circumstances, most jurisdictions will recognize a person's unfitness to plead. Psychiatry has also been used to classify non-conformance as mental illness; for example, to stifle political dissent in totalitarian regimes, as documented by dissenting authors such as Alexander Solzhenitsyn.

The distinction between psychiatry used for treatment or for punishment, is ethically important. I was involved in advising a Victorian Government Minister about decisions about a well known violent prisoner. The government wanted him classified as mentally ill so that he could be incarcerated indefinitely in order to protect himself and others. The prisoner was not considered by the assessing psychiatrists to be insane, but to have an anti-social personality. He had been convicted of a 1976 armed robbery, in 1977 of threatening to kill (police), in 1978 of discharging a firearm in public, and in 1980 of three counts of attempted murder. He had often self-mutilated, including having:

- inserted a fishbone in his eye
- swallowed battery acid, brass polish, razor blades, wire and glass
- slashed his arms, chest and stomach 26 times with razor blades, tin and glass.
- cut both his ears
- injected urine
- drained a litre of his blood with a fountain pen
- inserted a razor blade in his anus
- cut off parts of his penis (twice) and scrotum
- inserted wire and staples in his urethra
- slashed his legs six times
- severed his Achilles tendons, cut off his heel, and nailed his feet to floor.

Unable to have him classified as mentally ill, the Victorian Parliament (in Australia) eventually passed the *Community Protection Act* 1988 to keep him in custody after completing his sentence on the grounds that he remained a "danger to community." He subsequently died in 1992 of peritonitis after further self-inflicted abdominal wounds with a ball point pen.

4.7 Families and Confidentiality

The issue of confidentiality often arises in mental health. I was asked for advice about a patient, a woman aged 25 who had repeatedly self-harmed, feared abandonment, was possessive of relationships, though very capable in a structured work environment, and reluctant to talk about her childhood.

Her mother was also being treated in the same unit for stress. The mother disclosed an abusive husband, and the treating psychiatrist strongly suspected past sexual abuse of the children by the husband. The issue was that the information about abuse could not be disclosed to the daughter without violating the confidence of the mother. The two women had to be managed independently for fear of breaching privacy of one or the other.

In most jurisdictions, there are legal obligations to mandatorily report if a child or young person is at risk of continued abuse, but this situation involved past abuse of people now adults.

Confidentiality is not an absolute obligation. There are limits to it such as when someone endangers someone else, or even poses a danger to themselves. For instance, a doctor treating a man whose wife had left him, and whose adult children had little to do with him, left the consulting room in a state of mind that concerned his GP. She contacted police later in the day and asked for a safety check. On visiting the man's house they found him engaged in setting up a vacuum cleaner hose connecting the exhaust with the cabin of his car. The latter is something that has been made more difficult by design changes to exhausts in recent times. Later he was very grateful for the intervention.

5. Being a Patient

5.1 Love, Empathy and Suffering[1]

Philosophers are often perplexed by the problem of suffering, though at the same time, contemporary philosophers may appreciate, as the stoics did, the sense in which suffering can cause growth. The heroism of enduring suffering and gaining strength through that endurance is much appreciated by our community, even though not much sought at a personal level. Most of us are cowed by suffering, fearful of it and demanding of the technology to relieve it.

As a philosopher I see it as my task to try to understand the human condition, but as a believer my understanding is informed by Revelation, by the *imago dei*, and, in the light of that revelation, the idea of a Trinitarian anthropology. As a philosopher it is worth testing those matters of faith as stand alone propositions and not just as a mater of faith. An important work in that regard is Edith Stein's treatment of the concept of empathy, to which I will return.

Christians have traditionally understood that suffering can be an agent of growth through breaking down the effects of sin (II Cor. 4:7–18; Rom. 7), so that the life of Christ can be "manifested" or revealed through the believer. This process is seen as important for victory over the power of sin (Rom. 7:24), and for effectiveness in ministry (II Cor. 4:12).

Central to our understanding of the role of suffering is the life, death and resurrection of Jesus. The effects of sin have been conquered by the redeemer. His suffering has significance for us and through him our own suffering has significance. (Rom. 4:25; Rom. 6:1–11; Lk. 9:22–24; Jn. 12:24 Rom. 8:13; II Cor. 1:4–9; Phil. 3:10–11; I Pet. 4:1).

---

1 This paper was delivered as the 16th Fr. Francisco del Rios Memorial Lecture at the Faculty of Medicine and Surgery, University of Santo Tomas in Manila, February 1st 2007.

Believers hold that the major effects of "sin" in the sense of the sin of Adam and Eve are death and separation from God. That separation from God is not total, but from the human side our relationship with God is significantly marred. In Christ's death and resurrection these two principal effects are overcome. Death has lost its sting. Our lost humanity has been restored. It is now possible for us to begin the process of sanctification which leads to eternal life and ultimately to the Beatific Vision. However, the other "effects of sin" (2 Cor 4: 7–18), are still to be experienced. We still suffer even though we have been redeemed. But we are now able to deal with these "effects" of sin in the context of God's love. The link between sin and suffering, in the sense of actual sins committed as distinct from Original Sin, is contingent. John 9:1–3 makes it clear that the blind man's blindness is not the consequence of his or his parent's sin. It is connected with the Fall of Man and also with the idea of innocent suffering (vid. Job). However, that unmerited suffering is an opportunity for the display of God's goodness.[2]

Suffering is also seen as a source of wisdom, strengthening faith, or deepening our understanding. One who has trusted God in the midst of suffering has experienced faith at the deepest level (Phil. 4:10–12; Job; Rom. 5:3–5; Jas. 1:2–5; II Cor. 1:4; I Pet. 1:6, 7).

Suffering gives purpose to medicine. The cry of those in need draws a human response – to comfort, to relieve pain and distress, to sustain and to restore function. That human response is an expression of the human calling to love. It is a shared humanity. For the believer, though, there is the added dimension that this is a human life that is called to communion with God. Our human response then also is a witness to God's love, the love that Jesus manifest when he healed both physically and spiritually. The Christian physician remains ever conscious that his patient has an immortal soul and that suffering has a meaning which finds expression in human love.

---

2 Rev Dr John Fleming, personal communication 24/1/07.

Crucial to our understanding of suffering is the fact that we are embodied. Human bodiliness participates in the imago Dei. If the soul, created in God's image, forms matter to constitute the human body, then the human person as a whole is the bearer of the divine image in a spiritual as well as a bodily dimension. This conclusion is strengthened when the christological implications of the image of God are taken fully into account.[3]

In the words of the Vatican II, "In reality it is only in the mystery of the Word made flesh that the mystery of man truly becomes clear… Christ fully reveals man to himself and brings to light his most high calling"[4]

Christ's suffering is thus pivotal in our understanding of the place of suffering in our lives, the meaning of suffering and the fact that its existence is not a challenge to divine benevolence. The question, "Why do the innocent suffer?" is answered in the person, the life, death and resurrection of Christ. It is not God's will that we suffer, but the effect of sin from which he came to redeem us. The simple answer to the mystery of suffering is that it is a consequence of the exercise of free will, the same free will that makes us capable of love.

The call to grandeur and the depths of misery, both of which are a part of human experience, find their ultimate and simultaneous explanation in the light of revelation.[5] The human vocation is toward happiness, but we need also a theology of the opposite of happiness – suffering. Part of this puzzle is explained when Jesus responded to the question "Rabbi, who sinned, this man or his parents, that he would be born blind?"[6]

Jesus answered in a way that shows a dynamic relationship between love and suffering, "It was neither that this man sinned, nor his parents; but it was so that the works of God might be displayed in him."

---

3 International Theological Commission *Communion and Stewardship: Human Persons Created in the Image of God*, Vatican 2002.

4 *Gaudium et Spes*, n. 22.

5 *Gaudium et Spes*, n. 13.

6 John 9:2-3.

That prompts the question, could there be happiness if there were not also the possibility of suffering?

Jesus in the Beatitudes names suffering as the path to the Kingdom (happiness) – poverty, affliction, mourning, hunger, thirst, persecution and calumny.[7] Servais Pinckaers describes suffering as the concrete shape of the problem of evil.[8] Moral values are a response to suffering. Suffering and evil are the crucible from which knowledge of goodness shines forth. Evil is the absence of goodness.

In himself and in his healing works, Jesus took many opportunities to show us his goodness, his love.[9] In love, suffering finds dignity. Love gives meaning to suffering.[10]

There is a distinction to be drawn between a secular understanding of suffering and a Christian understanding. For the faithful believer, suffering is not cause for despair, but rather the occasion of hope, and it draws a response of love.

I find suffering perplexing. Suffering diminishes, thus the idea of growth through suffering is something of a contradiction.

Suffering diminishes a person by reducing and even removing the capacity for rationality that is the distinguishing characteristic of a human being. The romantic idea of the saintly hero or heroine uttering paeans of praise and thanksgiving, as her flesh burns or he is strangled by his own weight on the cross, is not my experience of suffering. Rather suffering tends to reduce us to that which is instinctual and animal as our bodies revolt against it, our reason takes flight and our capacities become limited by disability. The opposite of suffering is joy, peace and reason. Suffering attacks all three.

In recent times I have had occasion to seek comfort in Mark's account of the death of Christ. His cry, "My God, My God, why have

---

7 Matthew 5, Luke 6.

8 Pinckaers, Servais OP, *The Sources of Christian Ethics,* Catholic University of America Press 1995.

9 Pope John Paul II, *Dives in Misericordia,* n. 17.

10 Pope John Paul II, *Evangelium Vitae,* n. 97.

you abandoned me?"(Mark 15:34) has puzzled me as it has puzzled many others. To me this was an expression of the effects of extreme suffering, but did Jesus as God fully experience human suffering? Jesus' cry could not have been a cry of dereliction, despair and spiritual separation from the Father. That would be sin and Jesus could not have sinned.

The Catechism explains that Christ, having taken on humanity with all its sins, even though He Himself did not sin, makes the cry on behalf of sinful humanity. Nevertheless, having established Christ's solidarity with sinners, God "did not spare his own Son but gave him up for us all" so that we might be "reconciled to God by the death of his Son".[11]

St. Justin the Martyr claims[12] that the final cry of Jesus is the *purposeful* invocation of a psalm, denoting an act of prayer and implying a claim to prophetic fulfilment, and this view was taken up by many others including Irenaeus, Athanasius and Jerome.[13]

> "My God, my God, why have you forsaken me?
> Why are you so far from helping me, from the words of my groaning?
> O my God, I cry by day, but you do not answer;
> And by night, but find no rest."[14]

The Psalm then becomes an expression of praise for God. Thus the reference to the Psalm is an expression of praise for the Father, of connectedness and prophetic fulfilment, rather than of despair and spiritual disconnection. Jesus' invocation of the Psalm would thus be, as all his acts were, an expression of his boundless love, even in extremis and in agony.

---

11 *Catechism of the Catholic Church* n. 602–3.

12 Dialog*ue with Trypho* c. 97–99 in *Justin Martyr's Dialogue with Trypho* edited by RPC Hanson, Butterworth Press: London 1963 pp. 56–9.

13 White, Thomas Joseph, "Jesus' Cry on the Cross and His Beatific Vision", *Nova et Vetera*, Vol 5, Issue 3, Summer 2007 pp, 555–582.

14 *Psalm* 22:1–2.

In my own contemplation of Jesus' final cry, I have felt that it is important that Jesus' cry be understood as a reflection of his humanity. For Jesus as man, it would not have been human suffering if it did not humanly diminish him. My experience of suffering is that it suppresses capacity to reason. It reduces function. I wonder whether in his human suffering Jesus too experienced that loss of self, noting also that his cry was also an expression of his relationship to the Father.

Sometime ago, I suffered some complications of chronic heart disease. I had already had bypass surgery and recovered, when a chronic inflammatory disease caused inflammation of heart and lung tissue. While being taken to hospital by ambulance my condition worsened, I was in great pain, and my heart and lung function were affected. In the ambulance they were debating whether to give me a morphine infusion or adrenaline. Uppermost in my mind was to have the pain relieved. The paramedic dropped the morphine and stood on it making it unusable. They had stopped the vehicle so that both officers could attend to me. My wife who had been following by car, came to the window and as a doctor asked if she could help. I thought then, as I have on several other occasions, that I might be dying. I wanted to reassure Mary, but could not speak. Afterwards when I reflected on what happened, I was disappointed that I had not been capable of prayer. Confronted by the prospect of death, I just wanted the pain to stop. All the beautiful prayers, all the meaning to which I have tried in my life to give practical witness, deserted me at the moment when they should have been uppermost in my mind as I faced death.

On reflection, therefore, I take great comfort from the cry that Jesus gave. Rightly or wrongly, for me it represents his humanity in his capacity to suffer and to experience the incapacity that suffering brings. His cry seemed to me to signify the human loss that extreme suffering can cause. Nonetheless, his cry is perplexing for theologians because it reflects human suffering in one who, according to St. Thomas,[15] at all times possessed the beatific vision. It is perplexing

---

15 See Aquinas, *Summa Theologiae* III, q. 9, a. 2; q. 10, aa. 1–4.

Care of the Sick and the Dying

because it reflects the mystery that Christ as God is omniscient but as man can suffer, even this type of suffering which seems to indicate the solitariness of suffering. His final cry expresses the solitariness of suffering in his desire for the Father.

Jesus' cry also has significance because it testifies to both the separateness of the persons of the Blessed Trinity and their relationship to one another. In dealing with this topic, I particularly want to focus on Trinitarian Anthropology and to try to develop a fuller understanding of the nature of suffering and of its companions of hope and love.

When I found myself suffering and unable to communicate, I recall two very strong desires. One was to be free of the burden of pain. The other was to be able to reach out to Mary to both reassure her and to receive the comfort of her nearness and support. These desires were related. Somehow reaching out to her would relieve my suffering. Somehow I needed and wanted her nearness, not just that I expected death and wanted to say farewell, but simply I wanted her with me.

A puzzle for me is that despite being confident intellectually in my relationship to God, despite my prayer life and the great gift of prayer, in that moment it was to Mary, rather than to God that I turned.

But the fact that it was another that I sought seems both very human and very Christ-like. In his agony, it seems, Jesus humanly cried out to the Father presumably seeking, expecting, hoping for his presence, his nearness.

My failure to similarly seek the Father reflects my human imperfection. That I wanted to call out to Mary does however indicate her importance to me in the desire for her to be with me at that moment that I thought might be a moment of transition from this life. This has led me to reflect upon the humanly limited parallel that there is between persons in marriage and the persons of the Holy Trinity.

In this I want to express caution. The idea of marriage as expressive of Trinitarian love, has not been uncontentious. It is, after all, a view that was rejected by St. Augustine. In *De Trinitate*, he rebukes those who purport "to discover the divine image of the Trinity in a trinity of persons which belong to the natural human order: an image which would be realised in marriage by the presence of man, woman and child."[16]

However, despite Augustine's rebuke, Pope John Paul II in his Letter to Families writes,

> "Human fatherhood and motherhood, while remaining *biologically similar* to that of other living beings in nature, contain in an essential and unique way a *"likeness" to God* which is the basis of the family as a community of human life, as a community of persons united in love (*communio personarum*).
>
> "In the light of the New Testament it is possible to discern how *the primordial model of the family is to be sought in God himself*, in the Trinitarian mystery of his life. The divine "We" is the eternal pattern of the human "we", especially of that "we" formed by the man and the woman created in the divine image and likeness."[17]

I am venturing into stormy waters, but I am inclined to think that this difference between John Paul II and Augustine reflects a difference between Plato's rationalism and Aristotle's empiricism, a difference that is then reflected between Augustine and Thomas.

As a Platonist, Augustine represents the view that knowledge is a priori (comes before experience) and that is reflected in Augustine's notion of the immateriality of the intellect. It is too simplistic, but one might say that for Augustine, God is central and unity is obtained by rejection of the material and thus coming closer to God. For Thomas Aquinas, the Aristotelian, knowledge is a posteriori (comes after experience). Thus for Aquinas the human person is a unity of form and matter made in the image and likeness of God. We can then

---

16 St Augustine, *de Trinitate XII. V.5 Corpus Christianorum Series Latina 50 (1968)* pp. 359–60 *cf.* Marc Cardinal Oellet *Divine likeness: Toward a Trinitarian Anthropology of the Family* Michigan: Wm. B Erdmans 2006, p. 21.

17 John Paul II Letter to Families (1994) n. 6.

attempt to understand God through understanding man as form and matter within the imago dei.

Also too simplistically, following Augustine, we can seek to understand man by understanding God and, following Aquinas, we can seek to understand God by understanding man. John Paul II, by encouraging a Trinitarian Anthropology takes us in both directions. We can seek to understand ourselves as men and women through understanding the Trinity, but we can also try to understand the Trinity through our experience as men and women made in Their image and likeness. In my own weak way, I am proud of my own desire for Mary's nearness and her empathy, even though I do not profess to understand why her nearness should be so significant to me. But my frustration is that my cry did not include the sentiment of Psalm 130, the *De Profundis*, which I have recited as others neared death and have hoped would be the wish that I would express. Why was my appeal for Mary and not for God?

I recall a family moment several years ago when Mary and I were at Mass with one of our sons, then thirteen. Unusually, instead of a sermon, our priest asked us to complete a survey that had been endorsed by the Australian Bishops. The survey was part of some research into the faith and practice of the faith of attending Catholics. One of the questions we were asked was who was most important to us. Our son, who was watching each of us, was horrified that we both had written that God was the most important person in our lives. Naturally, with a child's ego-centredness, he thought that he was far more important to us than someone whom, as he said, we had never met. What a shock it was for him. Even more of a shock was the news that after God, we ranked each other as next in importance. He has three siblings and began to wonder if in fact he came a distant sixth in the race for our love!

His puzzle though is a more of a puzzle for me than I would have thought for, when tested, like Peter perhaps, it was not God whom I found myself desiring but Mary.

Even more perplexing though is the desire for her empathy. The desire for empathy is a puzzle. Sympathy is more understandable.

We can want someone to understand how we feel and even that they feel the same way about something. It is a sense of fellowship and community. But to desire that someone should actually experience our feeling, our pain, our joy, our love is something else. Why would we want them to suffer, if we love them?

Suffering is both solitary in that only I experience my suffering, but through empathy it can cause the suffering of another. One only has to consider the anguish of a parent of a child who is suffering. In my work with teenagers with cancer, it often struck me that the suffering of the parents was greater than the suffering of the child who actually experienced the illness. More than that, often it is the dying child who leads the parent in acceptance and understanding.

One can understand a desire of a spouse to shield the other from one's own suffering, to make light of it, to withhold the truth. But equally, one can understand a desire for empathy. It is a desire not just for community, but for unity.

Blessed Edith Stein writes on the importance of empathising with another. It is through that engagement that we come to a deeper understanding of our own psychic reality.[18] The desire for empathy, is a desire for understanding. Suffering is a moment not just for growth in oneself, in a stoical sense, but through empathy it becomes a moment of mutual growth as the "I" becomes "we".

A puzzle for a married person is that, as human beings made in the image and likeness of God, our vocation is to love God. We are called to communion with him. But our vocation in this life is to give ourselves completely in love for our spouse.

A celibate may give him or herself to God in witness to the life that is to come of perfect union with God, but a married person is called to express that love in union with another.

In recent times, some who have been inspired by Pope John Paul II, have considered the relationship between the persons of

---

18 Stein, Edith *On the Problem of Empathy* Washington: ICS Publications 1989, pp. 88–9.

the Holy Trinity as a model for the relationship between spouses. The basis for such a thought is in part consideration of the imago dei, the fact that we are made man and woman, each in the image and likeness of God, and, of course, the fact that Christ described himself in terms of the marital relationship, the bridegroom and the Church as bride. The marriage relationship is also described as a covenant modelled on the covenant between God and his people, and finally we have the image of Christ's own suffering and death on the cross as a model for human love, including the love that spouses have for one another.

All this points to the essential holiness of the marriage relationship and its capacity to be an avenue for expressing the imago dei. Through marriage we can aspire to the perfection of a love that is truly expressive of being made in the image and likeness of God, and marriage is a relationship that Jesus used to describe himself. As Pope Paul VI expressed it, "…husband and wife, through that mutual gift of themselves, which is specific and exclusive to them alone, develop that union of two persons in which they perfect one another, cooperating with God in the generation and rearing of new lives." In this, it seems, Paul VI gave the first authoritative recognition that couples could seek perfection through their relationship. In fact, I found in some of the manuals in use in the first half of the last century, this view was described as heresy.

As Christians, we well understand marital love as the willingness to endure suffering for the other, the complete gift of self, and the overpowering idea of imitating Christ's gift on the cross in that giving. John Paul II describes the family as the environment in which man can exist for himself by the unselfish gift of himself.[19]

A puzzle for me is the place of empathy in marital love. If I am suffering, I draw strength from the presence of my spouse. I want her with me, just as I would want to be with her if she were suffering. But how is it love to want her to be part of my suffering?

---

19 Letter to Families n. 11.

Ultimately, we are helpless to prevent our own suffering or the suffering of a spouse. Suffering, illness, loss of capacity through disease or simply ageing, and finally death are facts of human existence. But that suffering is ameliorated by love. In some way, by participating in the love of another, we seem to participate in God's love. In the person of the other, and the communion of persons that we form with another, we encounter Divine love.

In his dying Jesus calls for the love of his Father. My own experience of spousal love at a moment of suffering and in expectation of death, seem to provide some insight into a possible understanding of the nature of the cry. Looking at it from the opposite direction, Jesus' cry seems to indicate his need for empathy, his need for the presence of the Father in his suffering.

As spouses, though, we are helpless to prevent the end of our relationships through death. Dying separates us. The relationship between spouses is thus not a substitute for a relationship with God. But the gift that God gave to Adam and Eve was the gift of love, a gift that humanly introduces God's love to them. In the persons of one's spouse is the nearness and intimacy of God and the capacity for a communion of persons which is ultimately our vocation. Our spousal love leads us to God by giving us the opportunity for love that ultimately is love for God, and in empathy we can be united to the other in the way in which we hope ultimately to be united with God.

In *Lumen Gentium* the idea is expressed that through the sacrament of marriage, couples signify and share in the mystery of the unity and fruitful love between Christ and the Church.

> "The description of sacramental grace of marriage allows us to catch a glimpse of the fact that the spouse's mission goes far beyond the natural order of procreation and education of children. A certain classic representation of this grace tended to describe it exclusively in function of nature, emphasizing the perfection of nature and its ends as all there is to say about sacramental marriage. However, Vatican II underlined more the personal dimension of

> the sacrament and of conjugal love. It expressed sacramental grace in terms of an encounter with Christ and a consecration in the Holy Spirit "...so our Savior, the spouse of the Church, encounters Christian spouses through the sacrament of marriage. He abides with them..."[20]

As Marc Cardinal Ouellet expresses it, "by their marriage, every couple marries Christ". Death then is not an end to the gift of love given in marriage, rather it is the fulfilment of the vocation of marriage, the call to love God. The love of one's spouse is the love of God in whose image one's spouse is made.

One of my daughters when she was of pre-school age took part in a nativity play. We watched her proudly as, dressed in a white dress, veil and wings, she waited with the other angels for their turn to enter the scene. The time came and she began her demure walk across the stage, hands held in prayer before her and head piously bowed. When well across the stage she realised that the other angels, stage struck no doubt, were not following her. She turned to them and with a voice better suited to the playground shouted, "Come on", and waved them towards her. In our household since, when asked to do something, my response is often to say resignedly, "You have the voice of an angel". It seems always to be the case that angels are sent to tell people to do things.

There is some parallel in this to the gift of a spouse. I guess were it not for the fall, we would have had no need for angels. But in the state in which we find ourselves, the notion that the love of one's spouse is the love of God has many resonances. The particular resonance that motivated this paper is the desire for empathy and its significance in understanding human love in the context of human suffering.

The cry of love is a cry for communion. When a frustrated lover stands alone bewailing his fate, his solitary pain is not necessarily the

---

20 Oellet, Marc Cardinal, *Divine Likeness: Toward a Trinitarian Anthropology of the Family*, Michigan: Wm. B Erdmans 2006, p. 130.

unhappiness of she who for whom he hopes. Rather it is his own unhappiness, his own lack of opportunity to give and receive love.

We reason with him, telling him to move on, to find another because his affections are misplaced. She does not reciprocate. But he, in lover's grief, finds no consolation in that advice. In his mind she is not substitutable. There is an element of comedy in that situation, because there has been no mutual gift of self. But when a man similarly cries for the nearness of his spouse in his suffering, and she is unavailable, that is not comedy but tragedy. My grandmother, Nancy, recalls arriving at St Vincent's Hospital to hear the cries of her dying Italian husband, Ercole, "Nensi, Nensi, Nensi…"[21]

If in his suffering, a husband were to say, do not inform her, as I do not want her to be with me in my suffering, that too would seem to be tragedy. Yet it seems quite rational to say, I do not want her to suffer simply because I am suffering. That prompts me to ask whether there is gift to another in calling on her to be near in one's suffering.

One can certainly understand how deeply she would be likely to resent being deprived of the opportunity to be with him in his suffering. It would not be a consolation to her to say, "But I did not want you to suffer because I was suffering". She may well feel a lack of love in the exclusion, and no benefit at all in her being left in peaceful ignorance. The sacrament of marriage is unity. The gift of love is not one-sided but mutual. It is a oneness that transcends the bonds of friendship. It confers a right for her to be with him in his suffering. For him to wish to leave her in peaceful ignorance would have violated that unity. He does not have a moral right to that solitariness.

Were he to say, "I preferred to be alone with God in my suffering," would that have justified the exclusion? I would think it would not. The nature of the sacrament includes Christ, but in and through the relationship. Jesus does not replace the spouse in the relationship. He is loved in the person of the spouse.

---

21 Beeching, Ann, *Nancy Takes the Stick: An Autobiography of Contessa Filippini Australian opera pioneer 1896–1987,* published by C. Tonti-Filippini, NSCAN Technologies: Melbourne 1988.

This has been a very personal reflection and obviously every married person will have a unique experience of the spousal relationship. However it does seem to indicate that while believers hold that every member of the human family is called to communion with God, and every member of the human family is made in the image of God, and has the model of communion of persons of the Blessed Holy Trinity as the model for human relating, married persons are called to a spirituality that essentially involves the other. The other uniquely forms the bonds of empathy so that our spirituality becomes not "I" but "we".

With the other we express our union with the Divine. With the other we find not only empathetic joy, but also empathy in suffering as we experience the trials and tribulations of this life, finding, in the spouse, the gift of the person of Jesus, and thus experiencing a unity that is not only an expression of our vocation to be in communion with the Holy Trinity, but expressive of the interpersonal communion that exists between the persons of the Holy Trinity. The final cry of Jesus to the Father seems to express both his solitariness in suffering and his desire for empathy and unity. That desire for empathy and unity is a model for the spousal relationship in our vocation to express our witness to a human nature made in God's image. That sharing in Christ Jesus in the person of the other enlivens each day of our lives together, especially through the joys and sorrows of love, companionship and parenting, but it has particularly poignancy as we face diminishment through ageing and disease. Jesus as lover, as teacher, and as friend illuminates our lives, but it is Jesus on the Cross who brings us together in empathetic union with each other, just as he sought union with the Father.

5.2 Living with Disability and Chronic Illness

5.2.1 A Personal Note

This chapter is inevitably in part autobiographical, as my own experience of chronic illness informs my understanding of it. I am on a journey through chronic illness and increasing disability which I have described in volume one.

From time to time I am exposed to and affected by hospital-based infections. Most recently, I suffered double pneumonia for which I was hospitalised including two days in intensive care. While there I was asked by a senior physician whether I would like not to be resuscitated in the event of a cardiac or respiratory arrest. At the time my breathing was machine-assisted, and I was in a state of acute distress and struggling to keep my oxygen saturation levels at a reasonable level. It was both confronting and demoralising to be asked that question, at a time of acute illness, implying as he did by his question that my plight might be hopeless. The question is much more appropriate in a situation of advanced degenerative illness when resuscitation measures are unlikely to be successful, and frailness would make such attempts very burdensome. Even then, I was not really in a fit state at that time to manage his suggestion. Thankfully, I had previously completed some advice for end of life care which I gave to Mary and to my physician and have had included in my hospital notes (see last section of chapter). I referred him to that.

The narrative of our faith experience is such an individual journey. A friend who lives in our neighbourhood suffers from schizophrenia. He began a medical course years ago but dropped out and has been an invalid since, despite being quite brilliant. He comes to see me infrequently. Recently he told me that I would be a great mate if I were not so busy with my family and my work! I look at his circumstances, his suffering, and know that my problems just do not compare. I told him about this book and he said that he would be much more interested if I were to write about living with my illness – hence this very autobiographical chapter. But I am not sure that my narrative would be at all helpful to him. My work has allowed me a status and a place in life that is unfortunately denied him. His coping with illness requires far more courage and resilience.

We, as a community, do so little to find ways in which people who have a disabling mental illness can contribute. Often mental illness is episodal, and between episodes, so much more could be made available to them, than we currently offer, because we tend to classify people who have a mental illness by those episodes, and not by their peak functioning. It was a wonderful witness that the Hon Andrew Robb MP gave recently when he made public his own battle with mental illness.

5.2.2 The Mystery of Disability and Suffering

Crucial for a Christian philosopher is the belief in equal respect for every member of the human family. We believe that each one, no matter the level of disability, is made in the image and likeness of God and is called to communion with Him. Modern science tells us that that inherent capacity is because each member of the human family contains the human genome. From the moment that the first cell of the new being is formed, the genome within that cell directs the development toward embryogenesis, and directs the differentiation that results in the formation of organs including those important neural cells that mean that this being has the inherent capacity for loving, doubting, wondering and affirming. All that is needed is a favourable environment.

I remember when Brian Johns, who has Downs Syndrome, then about twelve and the son of my assistant Myrna and her husband Tom, picked up one of our children, then a toddler. He was so careful in the way he held her and the joy on his smiling face was so radiant. Everything about him spoke of love. At the time I had been reading a book by Susan Hayes about disability[22] which included a section on disability and parenting. She reported that people like Brian with cognitive impairment may be disabled in many ways, but if they become parents, their children do not necessarily suffer because of their disability. In fact their ability to give themselves in love may be superior to those of us with higher, normal intelligence quotients, but who may be too busy to give the care needed. Parents with cognitive disability may need help with parenting, but not necessarily with giving their children the love that is the core of what it is to parent successfully.

---

22 Hayes, S C and Hayes, R., *Mental Retardation: Law, Policy and Administration,* Sydney: The Law Book Co Ltd. 1982.

With Brian we may never know, because many with Downs Syndrome are also infertile. However there is not the slightest doubt he is made in the image and likeness of God, loved by God and able to love.

We all suffer from disabilities to greater or lesser extents at different stages of our lives. We entered life disabled, and it is likely that we will leave it disabled. Too often we speak of disability as a third person phenomenon when in fact we are talking about all of us.

One of the tasks I had for the National Health and Medical Research Council was to chair a committee to develop ethical guidelines for the care of people in an unresponsive or minimally responsive state. I have written about the experience elsewhere in this book. One of the disconcerting aspects of that experience was the view expressed by some theologians that people in an unresponsive state, (often the prejudicial term "vegetative state" is used) lack the capacity for friendship with God and therefore there is no benefit in acting to sustain their lives.[23] My view was that just as they are so often loved by their families, despite their disability, they too must still be loved by God. God's love is unilateral, not reciprocal, and so too should our love be.

I remember vividly that, at the launch of the guidelines, a young man who had been previously diagnosed with being in the unresponsive state, was in that state for two years, and had had a prognosis never to recover, did speak to us and thanked his parents (a doctor and a nurse) for their unfailing love and determination to keep supporting him no matter the medical advice about the futility of doing so.

Who are we to say who is worthy of God's love?

As a student I lived for a time in a shared household. They were wonderful young people and willing to accept into the household a friend of mine, Denis Cheesman, whom I had met and previously lived with at Mannix College at Monash University. Denis had advanced Friedrich's Ataxia, insulin dependent diabetes which was not

---

23 See for instance, O'Rourke, Kevin "Reflections on the Papal Allocution Concerning Care for Persistent Vegetative State Patients" *Christian Bioethics* (2006) 12 (1): 83–97.

well controlled, and he was almost quadriplegic, as well as gradually losing his sight, hearing and speech through the disease.

At that time Quality Adjusted Life Years (QALYS) were much in discussion. These were a way of assessing the benefits of treatment by assessing how much longer a person would live with treatment and at what quality, and then assigning a value that could be used to ration treatment and direct it to where it would produce the most benefit.

Dr Barry Catchlove, then CEO of the Royal Children's Hospital in Melbourne, had produced a set of questions to provide a quality of life rating as a score out of ten. The questions were mostly related to function. Denis scored a low 3/10 and the scheme recommended that life support be removed for scores of 4 or less.

We used to take Denis to Monash University each day, and leave him in the Union Building at what was known as the Small Café, which in fact was a very large café and a very common meeting point, if you could stand the constant strong smell of marijuana and tobacco smoke. These days, I guess smoking is banned in such places, but it was not then and there was also a belief (possibly untrue) that the Victorian Police paid no attention to the obvious trading in marijuana that took place in or around the café, because the University was Federal territory.

At the café, Denis would greet whomever happened to be passing and rely on them to hold his coffee, feed him, take him to the toilet (including all that was required) and wherever he needed to go. After completing his LLB, he used to enrol in a Master of Law each year, then defer, leaving him free to access the campus, attending the odd lecture, but not seriously studying, while attending student activities.

Denis used to say that he existed in order to give others the opportunity to be more human. There was a truth to that because, faced with his obvious need, we did all become more human at that usually very self-centred phase of life. Our own difficulties, whatever they were, paled into insignificance alongside his. He rescued so many of us, including me, by being so needy. Of course it was more than his neediness. He was so courageous, so cheerful, so engaging in his interest in each of us.

Disability is only comparative. Often it is those who are most able who are most in need of love, and often that means having someone to love as much as being loved. By being someone in need, Denis gave so much purpose and meaning to others.

Often people facing old age or illness talk about not wanting to be a burden to others when in fact so many people need someone they can help. Agape and eros, Pope Benedict tells us, are two dimensions of divine love: love of another and being received in love by another. God loves us (agape) and wants us to love him (eros).

Disability can cause great existential suffering, the suffering especially of loneliness. So many of us have a place in community and relationships through our employment. Too often disability robs people of that status and the social opportunities that it brings.

5.2.3 Existential Suffering

Existential suffering is a complex phenomenon. An aspect of it is the person's own sense of self worth and purpose and what they understand by love. One can see oneself as a burden, or one can see oneself as giving others the opportunity to express themselves in the love and service they give. If I understand my purpose in utilitarian or consequentialist terms, then the concept of what Ronald Dworkin calls a "narrative wreck"[24] has significance. There can be a life not worth living. If I understand that my life has meaning in the relationships of which I am a part, then I can accept that my role at this stage of life might be to accept dependence on others. Sometimes it requires love to accept the role of another and their giving. Sometimes it can be harder to receive than to give. Towards the end of life, it is usually necessary to accept that one has become incapacitated, to pass responsibilities to others and, for a believer, to prepare for the life to come, relinquishing those matters of this life that increasingly become less significant. The theological virtues of faith, hope and

---

24 Dworkin, Ronald, *Life's Dominion: An Argument About Abortion, Euthanasia, and Individual Freedom*, New York: Alfred A. Knopf, 1993.

love play a crucial role at the end of life. To a non-believer they might not make much sense, or at least not the same sense, and that may lead to the depressing conclusion that life as a burden, to oneself or to others, is a life that should not be lived.

As discussed in detail in chapter three, the discussion of euthanasia, and the passing of euthanasia legislation, promotes the idea of a life not worth living and places conditions upon love. We take meaning from those around us and, if euthanasia is an option, or is proposed as an option, then with it go a set of assumptions that undermine the individual's acceptance of what life brings, suggesting instead a responsibility to control life and to control its end. Knowing that those around us know that we could take the euthanasia option would greatly increase the likelihood of feeling that one is a burden, and should therefore put oneself out of their misery. Legalization of euthanasia is not just about individual freedom, it is about all of us, affecting all of us because it is about altering a fundamental premise of a caring, democratic society – that every member of the human family is of equal worth and dignity.

A significant factor for me would be that my doctors and nurses, on whom I depend not just for information and care, but also for their moral support, would be legally obliged to temper their support and advice, about what is best for my health, with advice that euthanasia or physician-assisted suicide is an option for me, and presumably information about how it might be achieved. That would utterly change the relationship from engagement in a common project of coping with illness to something quite different.

Chronic illness is often a struggle. It can have moments, especially during acute episodes, when continuing with treatment, on which life depends, seems not worth the struggle. Unsurprisingly, depression is an aspect of chronic illness and not helped by acute exacerbation of symptoms. Fewer responses could be more likely to fuel depression than one's doctor suggesting assistance so that one could quietly and comfortably suicide. It would be like a football coach of a bottom-side telling the players not to bother playing because defeat is inevitable.

"Who am I?" is a question that we all face and without love we may tend to answer it only in terms of achievement. When illness and disability reduce capacity for achievement, the question may have a very negative despairing answer. One may see oneself as defined by pain, illness and incapacity and by the burden one is on others, and even obliged to put one's miserable self out of their misery. So much depends on others and their attitudes, though ultimately the will to continue can only be one's own, and so much depends on one's view of the world and what gives life meaning. We do admire someone who continues to live life as fully as they can despite illness and disability. However, we need to be aware of the importance of the relationships that make that possible. It is very hard to do it alone. The relationships to health professionals and their unqualified commitment to the service of health is an important aspect of the patient maintaining confidence and positivity.

5.2.4 Being a Burden to Others

When confronted by someone who is in a state despair and feeling that they are a burden to others, a response one might make would be to seek to explore the person's relationships with their family and friends, to look around them for meaning and purpose.

The Order of Malta contributes to a biography project offered to palliative care patients. Volunteers undertake careful training to become biographers. They may then sit with a dying person, with their consent, asking pertinent questions, and with a recorder, so that they can accurately transcribe the written story of the person's life. It is a wonderful project that adds so much meaning to that stage of a person's life, both for them and for the family, because the systematic recovery of their personal history is always rich in purpose and meaning, and relationships. The process helps strengthen existing relationships, because it creates a sense of appreciation of who the person really is. The issue in someone feeling that they are a burden, is their perception that others may be feeling that way, wishing to be rid of them. That may be a false perception but it is a perception that is cultivated by our culture, especially its individualism and consequentialism. The biography project rekindles interest in whom the person is, not just the frail person nearing the end of life, but their whole life, the choices made, their loves and losses, the achievements and the failures. It is wonderfully rewarding for that story to be known to family and to others, perhaps the first time that it has been told in such detail, and with the effort to locate the chronology as well as possible, and, of course, to encourage family to support the narrative with images and other memorabilia. Care is taken for the written account to be exclusively the narrative of the dying person, not a joint family history.

The biography project is a wonderful way to counter or avoid despair at the end of life. It creates meaning by exploring the relationships of the past and of the present. It is one way in which it is possible to show someone, who may feel hopeless and burdened, that they are loved and appreciated.

I knew a man dependant on dialysis who had lived with a friend for years. When the friend died of cancer, he decided that the dialysis was just too burdensome and he decided to stop, after discussing it with his Parish priest. He was advised that he was entitled to refuse treatment that is so burdensome. He made the arrangements to give his possessions to the St Vincent de Paul society and disposed of the lease on the house, before going into hospital for his last illness as the renal failure took hold without dialysis. While in hospital, the care he received from the nurses changed his mind. He resumed dialysis and had then to try to reverse his earlier decisions and recover his property, etc. It struck me at the time how important that nursing care was. I have so often encountered nursing care that took little for granted, that looked beyond the routine of treatment to locate the person, as a person, not just as a patient.

The danger in health care is that, when you surrender your trousers, the universal indicator of being admitted to hospital, you might as well cross out "person" and write "patient". I recall visiting an Assisted Reproductive Technology clinic to keep an appointment with a gynaecologist for discussion of some regulatory issue. He clearly had a waiting room of women waiting, and I expressed discomfort at taking his time when he was so busy and causing them to wait longer. He responded along the lines of, "Don't worry! They are patients, they are meant to be patient." Having been a patient so often, I continued to feel uncomfortable.

It is not my place to advise a dependent elderly person who feels they are a burden to their carers. It may be my place to show my love and appreciation if it is welcome. When I worked at St Vincent's, in the security ward was an elderly multiple rapist, never to be released. He was the most complete misogynist that I have ever known. He simply hated women and thought his crimes against women justified because of the way his mother and a teacher had mistreated him. He was also a very sad man who was at that time likely to die of cancer. Sr. Claire, an elderly Franciscan Missionary of Mary, loved him and, despite his hatred of her kind, she gave his life purpose and meaning.

5.2.4.1 Some Effects of Faith

There is a major difference between believers and non-believers in the possession of the theological virtues, as discussed in volume one. For Christians, however, the dominant paradigm is the life, suffering and death of Christ, in which we accept suffering because there is love, and we identify our own suffering with Christ. Suffering draws a loving response. So, rather than seeing ourselves as a burden we are more likely to recognise the continued opportunities that we have for relationship. We also recognise that we have stewardship, but not ownership, of our bodies. It is not for us to decide that our life is to be disposed of.

I was involved with the drafting of the NHMRC *National Statement on the Ethical Conduct of Human Research*, but also a paired document that provided guidelines for the ethical conduct of research involving Aboriginal and Torres Strait people. A major difference was that the latter included a concept of reciprocity, so for instance a community might allow researchers to gather data provided that they funded a community centre. It was a significant cultural difference.

The basis of Christianity, and for that matter Judaism, is love of God and love of neighbour. We see personal fulfilment as dependent on making a gift of oneself to others. Love is unilateral in that we should give without counting the cost, even though we accept also that we desire to be loved. Agape, the desire to love, and eros, the desire to be loved are both part of God's love and therefore part of a Judeo-Christian understanding of human love. But agape and eros are not a reciprocity. We do not give love as a price for being loved. The two are not dependent on each other. Hence we can understand the unilateral nature of the individual commitments that are made in marriage – for better for worse, etc. In other words marriage involves mutual love, but each commits without conditions so that the commitment is permanent and exclusive – no matter what transpires later or whether the other party keeps to their commitment. It is not a reciprocal gift, but two mutual but unilateral commitments.

Christ used marital love on several occasions as an analogy for God's unconditional love for us. Christian love is not dependent on reciprocity. It applies also to parents. Parents usually love their children unilaterally – they love them no matter what they do or whether they return the affection. As a Christian, however, I am committed also to honour my parents and it makes no difference whether they are deserving of that love. I love them as those who gave me life, even if they were abusive or neglectful parents, which, happily, mine were not. Not to honour your parents, simply as parents, is to a large extent not to love who you are, because one's identity is so bound up with their identity. We share genetics and so much else. In our mothers, we have someone who carried us in the intimacy of that relationship for many months, and suffered through morning sickness, birth trauma and much else so that we could be born. For most, that is just the start of a lifetime of giving to us by both mother and father, but even if that is not so, they are irrevocably linked to our identity in being the origin of our lives. For many sons and daughters and their own children, the biography project reconstructs that origin and can be a significant moment of appreciating the sacrifices made.

As a parent and a spouse, my illness and disability are not just about me. I have a responsibility to contribute constructively to those several relationships, including how I cope with the illnesses and live life with my family despite disability. One contribution that a parent makes in to guide the next generation in how to cope with illness and dying.

My father died in 1987 after several years of treatment for non-Hodgkin's Lymphoma. Chemotherapy and its side effects were less controlled then and he suffered much through several periods of treatment, remission and relapse over a six year period. Living in the rural city of Bendigo, he was treated in Melbourne. He and my mother came to stay with me in Melbourne from time to time, first in a student house and then with Mary also, after we married. He was the perfect patient, uncomplaining, and doing exactly as advised. He belonged to a more stoical generation that did not complain or discuss emotions. During his last illness he developed secondary anaemia.

Being in the 1980s, the dominance of respect for autonomy and the requirement to inform was only beginning to influence what had been more paternalistic practices. I was hospital ethicist at St. Vincent's Hospital, where my father was a patient, and the oncologist was a colleague. For reasons best known to him the oncologist took me aside and told me that my father was dying. The red blood cell count was falling and they could not stop it. They were transfusing but losing ground. I asked him whether he had told my father and he said no. I asked if he would come with me when I went to tell my father, to answer his questions.

Reflecting on that time I know I did not handle that role well. I simply told him what I had been told, with no attempt to soften the blow. It came as a shock to my father. Later I came to know that one begins a conversation like that by focussing on the treatment being offered and what can be done. That was not my role. I ought to have insisted the physician talk about what they were doing, and then lead into the difficulties. After being told my unfortunately brief message, my father said, "I thought I was getting better". He had been of the view that if he did all that the oncologists asked, all would be well, despite having already suffered several recurrences after remission.

He started to breathe rapidly and shallowly and the oncologist asked him if he was having breathing difficulty. He replied, "No, I am upset". At 68, he had much life still to live and uncompleted projects. Nevertheless, soon after that initial shock, he indicated a straightforward acceptance of his dying, received the sacraments and died within three days of that announcement. In his last 48 hours, my mother did not leave him and two sisters of Charity, the late Srs. Christina and Brigid, maintained a death watch praying with her. When he breathed his last, several other members of the family and I were with my mother, saying the prayers for the dying. It was a very special time and some important conversations had been had between my father and individual members of the family over the three days in anticipation of his death.

I remember a moment while he was still lucid, when he asked the hospital chaplain whether the doctrine of purgatory was still "in". The priest replied, " Yes, and I think you are in it." Purgatory is indeed part of the Catholic tradition. It is the belief that those who die in a state of grace, a state in which they are open to God's love, but by no means perfect, can expect to be purified before achieving full communion with God. It is a very comforting doctrine, especially by those who may feel burdened by guilt and unworthy of God's presence. The priest's response was thus designed to give my father, a daily communicant in all the years I knew him, reassurance as he prepared to meet His Creator. It is a belief in a forgiving God. I remember saying the *De Profundis*, the very moving Psalm 130, "Out of the depths I cry to you, O Lord."

We were saying the Church's prayer for the dying as he began to breathe his last:

> Go forth, Christian soul, from this world
> in the name of God the almighty Father,
> who created you,
> in the name of Jesus Christ, the Son of the living God,
> who suffered for you,
> in the name of the Holy Spirit,
> who was poured out upon you.
> Go forth, faithful Christian!
>
> May you live in peace this day,
> may your home be with God in Zion,
> with Mary, the virgin Mother of God,
> with Joseph, and all the angels and saints . . .
>
> May you return to [your Creator]
> who formed you from the dust of the earth.
> May holy Mary, the angels, and all the saints
> come to meet you as you go forth from this life . . .
> May you see your Redeemer face to face

Whether he heard the words, I do not know, his breathing had ceased to be rapid and become slow and infrequent, usually associated with imminent death, but the timing was extraordinary. I wondered later whether it was providence, mere chance or the experience of those present to have elected to say that prayer then. As he died, Sr. Christina encouraged us to hold him. It seemed a strange thing to do: I do not recall ever having hugged my father. We were not physically affectionate.

Whenever I attended a baptism afterwards, and at the birth of our subsequent children, I recalled touching my father as he died, and I wonder at the similarity of transition from and into life. There are similarities in the combination of focus on breathing, trauma, grace and mystery, and finally peace.

I am grateful to my father for many things, but especially for his manner of dying. I pray that my own death may be as apparently accepting, peaceful and grace-filled as his seemed to be. In his illnesses and in his dying, he showed us how to live with illness and dying.

Of course those lessons do not happen suddenly, nor only at the time of grave illness. Preparing oneself and one's children for a good death is a matter of living for love. In the first instance parents display their unilateral love for their children and for each other. Children know that no matter what they do or what happens, their parents love them, and the relationship between the parents secures them in the richness of the depth of their unity, the fruitfulness of a love that is focussed outwards to give of itself, and for believers, living their faith by which they celebrate the joy of their love as a witness to the joyfulness of God's love. Truly spousal love seeks to demonstrate the same unilateral and unconditional aspects of divine love. Christian spouses are called to seek through their love to achieve perfection for their union.[25] They seek to make each other saintly.[26]

The role of a parent is to try to imitate God's unconditional love in which he gave us free will. As parents we nurture and protect for the day when the child gains the capacity to exercise that intelligent freedom that is his or her inheritance. In that process of nurturing a child together, the example of spousal and parental love is how we seek to prepare our children for the exigencies of life. However much we say to them and the use of so-called "quality time", it is in the practical realities of loving each other and loving them that we provide the most valuable lessons, despite our mistakes and imperfections.

5.2.5 Chronic Pain

I have written of the suffering of dependence, disability and illness. As well as disability and illness, there are those who suffer chronic pain. Pain is a strange phenomenon. Women experience extreme and often prolonged pain during childbirth, but that does not usually stop

---

25 Pope Paul VI *Humanae Vitae* n. 8; Pope Pius XI *Casti Connubii* n. 24.
26 This was expressed in a recent email exchange by Professor William E May from Washington October, 2011.

them from having another child. Suffering for a purpose is somehow different. People perform great acts of heroism including childbirth, choosing pain and suffering for higher ends. I recall being dumbfounded by a footballer completing a grand final with broken ribs that had caused a collapsed lung. Afterwards, he spent the night in intensive care.

The experience of pain is both a physical and a mental event. If it were just a mental event, one might control it, and by some accounts it is possible to do so by meditation, by mindfulness, and by self-hypnotherapy. However I have never been able to do so: the reality of anything other than minor physical pain usually defeats me eventually. One can manage well enough by concentrating (in my case on writing), but at some point fatigue robs us of those defences, and pain takes over. Knowing that it is chronic, may rob it of some of the anxiety that usually accompanies pain experience, but it remains what it is.

Medically, those who suffer from chronic pain are advised to manage their own pain because the use of pain relief is only a short-term measure. Sooner or later the body becomes so tolerant that the drugs simply do not work. Sooner or later, therefore, those with chronic pain have to rely on their own resources. It is a bleak reality, but nonetheless a reality.

There is a strange but perhaps necessary logic in pain clinics that insists on treating pain aggressively at its inception in order to try to prevent it becoming chronic pain. However once pain becomes chronic, the opposite occurs and they do their best to wean patients from pain relief. Being labelled with chronic pain is demeaning, because it implies a dependency on medical assistance and the problem of increasing tolerance, which in the minds of many is indistinguishable from drug dependency and addiction. It is difficult to be coping both with severe chronic pain, and the psychological warfare that is waged against those who are perceived to be addicted. There may also be physiological changes to the nerve pathways that can be part of chronic pain experience that increase sensitivity. That is a reason why pain is managed aggressively in the first instance to prevent that happening. There are different theories about how best to manage that circumstance and to what extent it is a reality. I was fortunate in the support I received from medical specialists who insisted on the reality of the sources of my chronic pain experiences, and their advocacy on my behalf, but I still felt the harsh judgements from some others and the awful experience of not being believed and of even being led to doubt myself. I am particularly grateful to my long term renal physician, Dr Andrew Tosolini.

5.2.6 Suffering and the Importance of Empathy

The existence of suffering is a challenge to faith. The problem of evil is not easily answered. How could a beneficent God permit so much suffering? That may be answered by saying that, in being made in the image and likeness of God, we have been given free will and the power to act freely according to our own reason, and that freedom includes a freedom to commit sin and thus cause evil. For God to take away our capacity to commit evil, would be to make us much less than we are. In fact without free will we would lack the very capacities that typify being human. Free will is necessary for us to be lovers.

That explanation accounts for much of the evil that we experience, but it is implausible to claim that all suffering is due to human activity. Human contributions may account to some extent for the natural disasters attributable to climate change, but hardly all such disasters and therefore all such suffering. Further, it simply is not plausible to say that all human illnesses are due to sin. In his *De Genesi ad Literam*, St Augustine suggests that one of the effects of sin and thus the Fall, was loss of understanding of our relationship to both God and nature.[27] Without that understanding, we live in disharmony with nature and suffer because of it. Thus if that were not so, if there

---

27 Augustine, *De Genesi ad Litteram 5.11.27* trans John Hammond Taylor as The *Literal Meaning of Genesis*, Ancient Christian Writers vols. 41–42, (New York: Newman Press, 1982). Vol 1.

were no sin, we would live in harmony with all creation, and we would not be in the path of the tsunami or the earthquake.

As I discussed in the previous chapter, when Jesus encountered a blind man he was asked by his disciples

> "Rabbi, who sinned, this man or his parents, that he was born blind?"[28]

They had assumed that such evil could only be the result of sin. Instead,

> "Neither this man nor his parents sinned," said Jesus, "but this happened so that the work of God might be displayed in his life. As long as it is day, we must do the work of him who sent me. Night is coming, when no one can work. While I am in the world, I am the light of the world."

It is a challenging response. But what it suggests is that suffering exists, not only as a result of sin, but, also, because it does have a purpose. There is a connection between love and suffering. It would be hard to understand love if we had never experienced suffering. The response of Jesus to suffering, both his own and that of others, through love, explains the connection between love and suffering. It is in our response to suffering that we give expression to the divine in us. By accepting our own suffering and responding with love to the suffering of others, we give witness to divine love.

To the Pharisees who challenged Jesus, he said:

> "For judgment I have come into this world, so that the blind will see and those who see will become blind." Some Pharisees who were with him heard him say this and asked, "What? Are we blind too?" Jesus said, "If you were blind, you would not be guilty of sin; but now that you claim you can see, your guilt remains."[29]

---

28 *John* 9: 1-5.
29 *John* 9:39-41.

Pain usually has a useful function in warning us that something is wrong and preventing us from doing further harm to ourselves. Sometimes however it no longer serves such a useful purpose, especially when it is chronic. Chronic severe pain as well as the suffering associated with disability, with mental illness, or with grief and loss, challenge our faith because they seem so purposeless. It seems difficult, when we experience such suffering, or see or experience the widespread suffering caused by natural events such as bushfires, earthquakes, tsunamis and floods, to accept that this is all necessary for the works of God to be displayed in us.

According to Pope John Paul II, suffering causes three emotions: compassion, admiration and fear.[30]

The suffering of another calls us to respond with compassion in order to assist the person. Compassion or empathy means to suffer with another. St. Teresa Benedicta of the Cross (Edith Stein) has written beautifully on empathy:

> The hand resting on the table does not lie there like the book beside it. It "presses" against the table more or less strongly; it lies there limpid or stretched; and I "see" the sensations of pressure and tension'. So far this example includes only the first level of accomplishment in empathy – the emergence of the experience of another. The second level involves delving into the content of the Other's experience. If this happens, then there is a movement from empathy as the passive association of our two lived bodies to empathy as the imaginative transposal of myself to the place of the Other:' my hand is moved (not in reality but "as if") to the place of the foreign one. It is moved into it and occupies its position and attitude, now feeling its sensations, though not primordially [i.e., not in the original] and not as being its own . . . the foreign hand is continually perceived as belonging to the foreign physical body so that the empathized sensations are continually brought into relief as foreign in contrast with our own sensations.[31]

---

30 Pope John Paul II, *Salvifici Dolores* 11 February 1984. n. 14–21.
31 Stein, Edith, *On the Problem of Empathy*, trans. Waltraut Stein, The Hague: Martinus Nijhoff 1964. p.54.

The effect of witnessing the suffering of another whom we love is a suffering of its own. Not the same suffering but somehow closely linked to it.

One of my children received some damage when a small brass bell was thrown by another, splitting his outer ear. The doctor administered a local anaesthetic so that he could stitch it. That involved several injections into the tissues of the ear on either side of the split. My son, showing immense control for an eight year old, allowed this to happen without complaint, but as I held his hand and with a hand on his shoulder I could feel that his whole body had become as stiff as board, his mouth tightly closed and his jaw locked, his expression blank and his eyes firmly fixed on some point on the ceiling. As a parent, I wished there was something more that I could do other than reassure him, and I felt in myself some of the tension that was in him to the point of feeling that I too was in pain. I felt similarly with the birth of each of the children while Mary grasped my hand, twisting my fingers as she endured the awful pain of the contractions. Childbirth is an experience beyond male imagining, but one who loves cannot help but be involved in the experience, however minimally.

Empathy is a strange phenomenon. As a young man, my contribution to the game of cricket was to try to bowl fast, not always accurately, but certainly with maximum effort. The action involves sprinting to the pitch and at full pace turning side on and delivering the ball from as high a position above one's head as can be managed to achieve bounce, then immediately stepping sideways so as not to damage the surface under the gaze of the ever observant umpire. It is a very unnatural action. The resultant twisting of the spinal column, shoulders and weight bearing joints under great pressure always caused pain. Even now, many years since I bowled a ball at pace, I cannot help but twitch and feel pain with each delivery when watching a Brett Lee, Mitchell Johnson or Shaun Tait – particularly the latter, who is a slinger as I was. Mary laughs at my very active couch life.

Human suffering often motivates us to respond to come to the aid of the other. Even the distant suffering of those affected by a natural disaster in another country evokes in us the desire to assist. Thus the emotion of compassion has an important role in connecting suffering and love, and the response gives meaning to the suffering by providing the opportunity for a relationship between those who suffer and those who respond.

We generally associate suffering not only with pain, but also with vulnerability, weakness and loss. When we see someone bear their suffering courageously, we usually experience a sense of admiration. As he aged and suffered illness, Blessed John Paul himself gave witness to the power and strength that may be a person's response to suffering. When Mary and I attended a meeting of theologians that he addressed on the topic of the unresponsive state in the year before he died, Mary wept when she saw his disability, the paralysis of one side and his effort to read the speech, which he did not complete. But at the end there was the same earnest desire to reach out to those in the room and physically touch them as he was wheeled between us. The suffering of heroes, particularly the suffering of Jesus on the Cross and in anticipation at Gethsemane, was for a purpose. Suffering thus provides the opportunity for achievement.

Our own suffering not only provokes compassion in others and opportunities for them to express their love, it also has a meaning in our endurance of it. We admire those who can endure great suffering for a higher purpose.

Suffering reminds us of our own mortality, weakness, and powerlessness. This can bring about fear as well, and may challenge our faith. Who has never, in the face of human suffering, calamity or misery, asked their God, why? It is one thing to fear death and what does or does not come after life. It is another to be rocked in your faith, and then to question God's love or even God's existence. A priest and mentor of mine, the late Fr Francis Harman, advised me to make my peace with God and not to wait until I was *in extremis* because one might not be able. I have on several occasions felt severe pain to the extent that I was unable to think rationally. I am most grateful to my wife, Mary, whose empathy at those times carried me across a sea of terror and near desperation, and through her love kept me close to God.

As mentioned earlier, in *Salvifici Dolores* the Holy Father speaks of an opportunity for those so challenged to undergo their own Gethsemane, their own Calvary, their own feeling of abandonment that hopefully and joyfully may lead also to their own conversion, their own resurrection and unity with Christ.

Christ's cry, "Eli, Eli. Why hast thou abandoned me," tells me of his humanity and his human loss of reason through pain such that, even as God, he could feel abandoned no matter that cognitively and as God he knew that could not be so. It also expresses his desire for the Father's love at that time of suffering.

Linking one's suffering to the suffering of Christ can give it redemptive effect. I know that the link made in prayer brings me closer to Him, and seems to make past sins insignificant. There is a dignity that I can feel, however undeservedly, through my acceptance of unavoidable suffering, sharing in the predicament of Job and of Jesus, finding their willingness to accept suffering inspirational in relation to my own.[32]

The importance of all this is the link between suffering and love. In response to our own suffering, the love of others for us may be expressed, and our suffering provides a context for understanding our closeness to Christ, in his acceptance of suffering for the redemption of humanity, and our own acceptance of suffering linked to His. Without human suffering and without Christ's suffering, there would be so much that we would not understand.

Without Christ's redemption of our sins, there would be so much not understood about faith and hope. In suffering pain, I have experienced hopelessness and despair, but I have also experienced the effect of Mary's love in carrying me through. She is a practical witness to the love of God, through which she exhibits the *imago dei* in her

---

32 Stuart, Paul, "Pope John Paul II and the Redemptive Power of Suffering", *AD2000*, May 2005 http://www.ad2000.com.au/articles/2005/may2005p20_1953.html.

person, and inspires faith and hope in that divine love when illness and disease attacks my person, and when it suppresses my capacity to respond cognitively, stripping away those features that so identify us human beings. Through Mary, I know God's love and can trust that God will carry me through, whatever befalls.

5.2.7 A Personal Response

Recently I was contacted by a man, a Catholic, who had been diagnosed with prostate cancer and contemplating surgery and other possible treatments. He expressed being unsettled and wanted to know his obligations with respect to treatment. At the time, I was convalescing after illness and hospitalisation and my own experience was very fresh in my mind. Amongst responses to some other queries, I wrote that I was sorry about his diagnosis, suggesting that it is a common diagnosis for older men but not very common in younger men of his age. Over 80% of men have a prostate cancer at death with most being undiagnosed and unrelated to the cause of death.

I explained that the Church takes the view that we should take good care of our health but that we do not have to use means that are overly burdensome. With each option for treatment that they offer, the medical team should explain the likely effects and the risks so that the patient can make an informed judgement about what he thinks is appropriate. At some stage a patient might say "enough, it is too burdensome", but that day may never come. Much depends on the kind of cancer involved. Some men have the surgery and are never troubled again. Some will need follow-up treatments.

In the first instance, I would simply pray to be in that first category and worry about other things, if and when they are raised and there may be further need for treatment. It may never happen.

It was not my place to start canvassing all the possibilities because much depends on what, in his case, they had discovered. But I did suggest that it sometimes happens that men are impotent for a time or even permanently, but I had no idea whether that might be a risk in his case. The best person to talk to about what to expect is the surgeon and, perhaps, the GP, who should receive a detailed letter about it from the surgeon. I went on to explain:

> Everyone at the hospital wants the best for you and if you do have prolonged oncology treatment you will get to know the oncology nurses. It is daunting to lose your trousers and become a patient but it has its good moments. Much depends on your own attitude to the staff. Questioning is always fine and you have every right to make your own decisions, but they also have much experience and, unless you perceive difficulty, it is usually best to go with the flow of what they recommend. If you do not understand it, is important to ask. Taking a notepad to consultations is fine as long as you explain that it is just for your own memory and so that you can better explain to your family. Otherwise they may see you as litigious and act more defensively. I try to have Mary along for consultations because I do not always understand it the first time and she can often correct me when I misrepresent what was said. It makes it much easier to discuss it later and it becomes a shared ordeal, not a lonely ordeal. I often feel she suffers more than I do for that reason.
>
> A man I am close to was diagnosed with prostrate cancer at age 58. He is schizophrenic and vulnerable and often not able to follow what is said. Having been asked to go with him, I took careful notes at consultations and tried to be there when there were significant events. He needed no other treatment and has been clear for six years. One time I remembered a painful procedure with some re-suturing of his wound – he was obese, which did not help, and the wound was large. Not knowing what else to do I laid my hands on his shoulders and he visibly relaxed. There is a role that someone close to you can play. There is little merit in trying to manage illness and treatment alone.
>
> Part of the difficulty for a first diagnosis of this nature is discovering a level of embodiedness that you may not have known. Your self image changes in being the one cared for and losing some pride, independence and machismo (for men).

However sick, I still try do the manly things as long as it is safe. Mary is very tolerant. I also found that with being off work and sick I could enjoy the family and Mary more. We have just had a lovely week, together all the time despite my illness – she took the time off. I have never felt more in love with her. The older children came home to cook for us and we had more time to talk. In earlier times when they were little I read to them while on dialysis treatment, especially at bed time, and admired their work and listened to the homework for the older ones. They were precious moments.

If you have to have chemo you might take your little child with you for at least part of the sessions, if they permit that. Lovely for both of you. Convalescing after surgery is another opportunity to read for them or hear their reading, watch their DVDs or tell them make up stories. Far from being a disaster it can be a great opportunity.

With my illnesses we found time to deepen our prayer life and Mary and I now say the evening office together before turning out the light. We seemed to be too tired and busy before. Saying the psalms together offers us so much and is often so apt. The pattern of prayer is very soothing and constantly affirms our trust in the Lord.

Illness need not be a disaster, just adaptation to change and making fresh discoveries about oneself and others. I have been on dialysis four times a week, four hours at a time for twenty years and have advanced heart disease for seven years including failed bypass surgery. I have lost some opportunities and had some bad things happen, but overall I would not change much. Mary and her love have been a constant, forever adapting but never at a loss.

You and your wife have much to endure but it is not all doom and gloom, just different and calling on you to place your trust in the Lord and your trust in your love for each other. You may be pleasantly surprised with what doors open that you did not know existed, including your own resilience and the depth and strength of your love for each other.

By the way, you are entitled to seek being anointed because you are sick and facing an operation. It is a very peaceful, very meaningful event. Just mention it to your priest.

5.2.8 Some End of Life Instructions

In relation to my own future care I have adapted the draft provided by the Catholic Health Australia[33] to my own circumstances.

1. I wish to be given appropriate care to preserve my life, and to cure, improve, or reduce or prevent deterioration in, any physical or medical condition I suffer.
2. I hold that death need not be resisted by every possible means. I ask that I not be given any treatment that, in the judgment of my senior available next of kin, after receiving medical advice, would not sustain, give comfort or treat me or relieve a condition I have, or would be overly burdensome to me or to others.
3. I ask that I be given adequate palliative treatments to manage uncomfortable or distressing symptoms, while maintaining, during the dying process, as much function as possible, especially lucidity. If it happens that the only way to manage my distress is with treatments that have the side effect of reducing lucidity or even shortening life, then I am prepared to accept these as foreseeable but not directly intended consequences.
4. I consider food (nutrition) and water (hydration) to be basic necessities. I wish to be provided with food and fluid for as long as I need them, intravenously or by tube, if necessary, and with other basic means of preserving my life and making me comfortable, unless or until such methods of treatment and care are ineffective in sustaining life or are overly burdensome to me or to others. However the burdensome nature of inserting or maintaining a tube is to be taken into account.
5. I understand that I am suffering from the following progressive illnesses: Renal failure, ischaemic heart disease, peripheral neuropathy, and rheumatoid auto-immune disease which causes inflammation including of the heart and lung.

---

33 Adapted from the Catholic Health Australia *Guide to Future Care Planning* approved by the Australian Bishops http://www.cha.org.au/site.php?id=223.

6. If I suffer from cognitive impairment to the extent that I can no longer understand the purpose of haemodialysis and this is a cause of distress I would want effective, non-burdensome treatment and care that is reasonably available to be continued, but would not want haemodialysis to be persisted with, if that decision was acceptable to my senior available next of kin.
7. I do not want my life to be ended by any action or omission that is directly intended to cause my death but recognise that withdrawing or withholding overly burdensome care is not such an omission as there are limits to the obligation to sustain life.
8. When it is thought that I am in the final stages of terminal illness or injury or that my death is imminent, I ask that all reasonable steps are taken to allow me to be with my family and reconciled to anyone from whom I may have become estranged, and that insofar as possible, I be allowed to die at home or at least in a home-like hospice or other institution if that is not overly burdensome to my family.
9. In my medical care, I wish to follow the rites and teachings of the Catholic Church. When I am approaching death I ask that I receive the appropriate ministry from a Catholic priest.
10. I wish to follow the teachings of the Catholic Church with regard to my medical care. I ask that the *Code of Ethical Standards for Catholic Health and Aged Care Services in Australia* (CHA 2002) and other official church documents quoted therein or issued since be observed in my care. When I am approaching my death, I ask that I receive the Sacraments of the Church.

5.2.9 Afterword

This volume has combined some personal experiences with some more formal material on the relationships between health care professionals and people who are dependant upon for care during sickness and in their dying.

There are obvious conflicts over issues such as: euthanasia and physician assisted suicide, best interests versus substituted judgement in representation, the doctrine of informed consent versus duty to inform and the right to refuse the treatment offered, individualism versus communitarianism, and justice versus utilitarianism and the use of QALYs. In volume one I discussed the theoretical differences. In this volume I wanted to offer a particular approach to the issues founded upon a Christian concept of love. That has taken me into areas that may be uncomfortable for someone who does not share my faith. Others who do share my faith may still have been uncomfortable with my particular approach to the distinction between faith and reason and other matters.

Whatever of those differences, what I wished to achieve was an offering to be considered alongside the many other voices on these issues. I have experienced the great joy and grace of finding love and faith strengthened by my experiences of illness. I pray that that process continues to be enriching, for I know how fragile the human experience can be. However, by giving these accounts of my experiences against the background of the debates in Bioethics over the nature of the relationships in healthcare, I hope that others may find something worthwhile, whether or not they agree.

Bibliography

Arango, Celso and Kahn, René "Progressive Brain Changes in Schizophrenia" *Schizophrenia Bulletin* 2008 March; Vol 34, No. 2, pp. 310–311

Augustine, St., *De Genesi ad Litteram 5.11.27 trans* John Hammond Taylor as The *Literal Meaning of Genesis*, Ancient Christian Writers vols. 41–42, (New York: Newman press, 1982). Vol 1

Augustine, St., *de Trinitate* XII. V.5 Corpus Christianorum Series Latina 50 (1968)

Australian Medical Council *Good Medical Practice: A Code of Conduct for Doctors in Australia* (2010) http://www.amc.org.au/images/Final_Code.pdf

Baume P, O'Malley E. Euthanasia: attitudes and practices of medical practitioners. *Med J Aust* 1994; 161: 137–145

Beeching, Ann Nancy Takes the Stick: An Autobiography of Contessa Filippini Australian opera pioneer 1896–1987, published by C.Tonti-Filippini NSCAN Technologies: Melbourne 1988

Berzoff, Joan, Silverman, Phyllis *Living with Dying* Columbia University Press: New York, 2004

Bolam v Friern Hospital Management Committee (1957) 1 WLR 583 *Rogers v. Whitaker* (1992) 175 C.L.R. 479, 489.*Woods v Lowns and Procopis* (1995) 36 NSWLR 344

Catechism of the Catholic Church St Paul's Publications 1994

Catholic Health Australia *Guide to Future Care Planning* approved by the Australian Bishops http://www.cha.org.au/site.php?id=223

Clark, Peter "Tube Feedings and Persistent Vegetative State Patients: Ordinary or Extraordinary Means?" *Christian Bioethics* Volume 12, No. 1, May 2006 pp. 43–64

Crown Prosecution Service, "DPP publishes assisted suicide policy" 25/02/2010 Accessed 26/12/10 http://www.cps.gov.uk/news/press_releases/109_10/

Eric D'Arcy "Healthcare is not an industry" *Bioethics Outlook*, Vol 22 No 3 September 2011

Dlugoborski, Waclaw, and Franciszek Piper, editors, *Auschwitz, 1940–1945: Central Issues in the History of the Camp* Five Vols. Oświęcim: Auschwitz-Birkenau State Museum

Drugs, Poisons and Controlled Substances Act 1981 sections 70(1) & 71AC)

Eiser, Arnold R. and Matthew D. Weiss The Underachieving Advance Directive: Recommendations for Increasing Advance Directive Completion *The American Journal of Bioethics* :: Volume 1 Number 4 2001 p. 1–5

Fagerlin, Angela and Carl E. Schneider "Enough: The Failure of the Living Will" *The Hasting Centre Report Vole 34* No 2 March-April 2004

Fleming, John and Nicholas Tonti-Filippini (ed.) *Common Ground? Seeking an Australian Consensus on Abortion and Sex Education* St Paul Publications: Sydney 2007

Guardianship and Administration Act 2000 (Qld)

Hayes, S C and R Hayes,. *Mental Retardation: Law, policy and Administration* Sydney: The Law Book Co Ltd. 1982

Hermina Dykxhoorn Accessed 24/12/10 from http://www.euthanasia.com/netherlands.html

Hudson Peter, Kristjanson Linda J, Ashby Michael, Kelly Brian, Schofield Penelope, Hudson Rosalie, Aranda Sanchia, O'Connor Margaret, Street Annette. (2006) A systematic review of the desire for hastened death in patients with advanced disease and the evidence base of clinical guidelines *Palliative Medicine* 20, 693–71

Hulls, Rob *Second reading Speech, Charter of Human Rights and Responsibilities* Bill 2006 http://www.justice.vic.gov.au/wps/wcm/connect/justlib/DOJ+Internet/resources/4/b/4b6ab080404a3ef9a149fbf5f2791d4a/Second+Reading+Speech.pdf

Hurst, Samia A, Alex Mauron "Assisted suicide and euthanasia in Switzerland: allowing a role for non-physicians *BMJ* 2003; 326 : 271, 1 February 2003

International Theological Commission *Communion and Stewardship: Human Persons Created in the Image of God* Vatican 2002

Justin Martyr's Dialogue with Trypho edited by RPC Hanson, Lutterworth Press: London 1963 pp. 56–9

Kilner, John Who Lives? Who Dies? Ethical Criteria in Patient Selection YUP 1984

Kissane, David W Annette Street, Philip Nitschke, 'Seven deaths in Darwin: case studies under the Rights of the Terminally Ill Act, Northern Territory, Australia,' *The Lancet*, 1998 Vol 352: 1097–1102

Klein, Rudolf "Lessons for (and From) America " *American Journal of Public Health* January 2003, Volume 93, No. 1, pp. 61–3

Komesaroff, Paul A. and Ian Kerridge "The Australian medical Council draft code of professional conduct: good practice or creeping authoritarianism" MJA Vol 190 No 4 16 February 2009 pp. 204–5

MacIntyre, Alasdair *The Tasks of Philosophy: Selected Essays*, Vol 1 CUP 2006

Mak, Yvonne Yi Wood and Glyn Elwyn "Voices of the terminally ill: uncovering the meaning of desire for euthanasia" *Palliative Medicine*, Vol. 19, No. 4, 343–350 (2005)

Mattson MP 2005; "Energy intake, meal frequency, and health: a neurobiological perspective." *Annual Review of Nutrition* Volume 25, pp. 237–60 http://nutrition.suite101.com/article.cfm/the_effects_of_dehydration#ixzz0lE4fAb4z

Murray, Suellen and Powell, Anastasia *Sexual assault and adults with a disability: Enabling recognition, disclosure and a just response* Published by the Australian Institute of Family Studies. Issues no. 9 2008

National Health and medical Research Council, *Ethical Guidelines for the Care of People in Post Coma Unresponsive or a Minimally Responsive State* Australian Government 2008 http://www.nhmrc.gov.au/_files_nhmrc/file/publications/synopses/e81.pdf

National Health and Medical Research Council, *National Statement on Ethical Conduct in Human Research* Australian Government 2007 http://www.nhmrc.gov.au/publications/ethics/2007_humans/section4.2.htm

National Health and Medical Research Council, *General Guidelines for Medical Practitioners on Providing Information to Patients* Australian Government 1993

Neuberger, Julia "A healthy view of dying" BMJ. 2003 July 26; 327(7408): 207–208

Newman, John Henry An Essay on the Development of Christian Doctrine Longman's Green and Co. London, New York and Calcutta 1909

NHMRC *National Statement on Ethical Conduct in Human Research* Australian Government 2007 n. 4.1.14.

Oellet, Marc Cardinal Divine likeness: Toward a Trinitarian Anthropology of the Family Michigan: Wm. B Erdmans 2006,

Organisation for Economic Co-operation and Development, *OECD Health Data 2006*, http://www.oecd.org/health/healthdata.

O'Rourke, Kevin "Reflections on the Papal Allocution Concerning Care for Persistent Vegetative State Patients" *Christian Bioethics* (2006) 12 (1): 83–97.

Pinckaers OP, Servais *The Sources of Christian Ethics* Catholic University of America Press 1995

Pope Benedict XVI, *Caritas in Veritate* Vatican City 2009

Pope John Paul II *Familiaris Consortio*

Pope John Paul II *Evangelium Vitae*

Pope John Paul II Address to an Internationakl Congress on Luife Sustaining Treatment and the Vegetative State Saturday, 20 March 2004 *http://www.vatican.va/holy_father/john_paul_ii/speeches/2004/march/documents/hf_jp-ii_spe_20040320_congress-fiamc_en.html*

Pope John Paul II *Dives in Misericordia*

Pope John Paul II *Letter to Families* (1994)

Pope John Paul II, *An address to an International Congress on "Life-Sustaining Treatments and Vegetative State: Scientific Advances and Ethical Dilemmas* Rome Saturday, 20 March 2004 Accessed from: http://www.vatican.va/holy_father/john_paul_ii/speeches/2004/march/documents/hf_jp-ii_spe_20040320_congress-fiamc_en.html

Pope John Paul II, *Evangelium Vitae* Vatican 25 March 1995, n. 65 Accessible from: http://www.vatican.va/holy_father/john_paul_ii/encyclicals/documents/hf_jp-ii_enc_25031995_evangelium-vitae_en.html

Pope John Paul II, *Salvifici Dolores* 11 February 1984

Pope Pius XII, "Address to 1st International Congress on Histopathology of the Nervous System" 14/9/52

Powers of Attorney Act 1998 (Qld)

Ratzinger, Joseph *In the Beginning..: A Catholic Understanding of the Story of Creation and the Fall* (English Translation) Our Sunday Visitor: Huntington, Indiana 1990

Reisfield GM, Wallace SK, Munsell MF, Webb FJ, Alvarez ER, Wilson GR. "Survival in cancer patients undergoing in-hospital cardiopulmonary resuscitation: a meta-analysis" *Resuscitation*. 2006 Nov;71(2):152–60. Epub 2006 Sep 20

Savulescu, Julian, "Conscientious Objection in Medicine." *BMJ* 2006 No. 332 pp: 294–297

Savulescu, Julian, "Should doctors practice according to their beliefs?" *MJA* 195 (9). 7 November 2011, p. 497

Saracci, Rodolfo "The world health organisation needs to reconsider its definition of health" *BMJ* 1997;314:1409 (10 May)

Scrutiny of Acts and Regulations Committee, Victorian Parliament *Alert Digests* http://www.parliament.vic.gov.au/archive/sarc/Alert_Digests_08/08alt11body.htm#Abortion_Law_Reform_Bill_2008

Smart, JJC "An Outline of a System of Utilitarianism Ethics," Ch 4 in Bernard Williams *Utilitarian: for and against* Cambridge University Press 1973

Stein, Edith *On the Problem of Empathy*, trans. Waltraut Stein, The Hague: Martinus Nijhoff 1964

Stuart, Paul "Pope John Paul II and the Redemptive Power of Suffering" *AD2000* May 2005 http://www.ad2000.com.au/articles/2005/may2005p20_1953.html

Taylor, Charles *The Ethics of Authenticity* Harvard University Press Cambridge, Massachusetts and London, England 1992

Ten, Chin Liew *Mill on Liberty* Oxford University Press 2001

Thomas Aquinas, St, *Summa theologiae* Translated by the Fathers of the Dominican Province Christian Classics: Maryland 1981

Tonti-Filippini, Nicholas "Blame Casemix: Not Just the Budget Cuts" *Quadrant* June 1995

Tonti-Filippini, Nicholas "Casemix is bad for patients" *Social Action* No. 147 February 1995

Tonti-Filippini, Nicholas (2000). *Human dignity: autonomy, sacredness and the international human rights instruments.* PhD thesis, Department of Philosophy, The University of Melbourne

Tonti-Filippini, Nicholas "Euthanasia and the Fragility of Living a Burdensome Life" *Nova et Vetera,* English Edition,Vol. 9, No. 3 (2011): 561–565

Tonti-Filippini, Nicholas "Some Refusals of Medical Treatment which Changed the Law of Victoria" *Medical Journal of Australia,* Vol 157, August 17 1992 pp. 277–9

United Nations *Convention against Illicit Traffic in Narcotic Drugs and Psychotropic Substances* http://www.unodc.org/unodc/en/treaties/illicit-trafficking.html

United Nations, *International Covenant on Civil and Political Rights.* http://www2.ohchr.org/english/law/ccpr.htm

United Nations, *International Covenant on Economic, Social and Cultural Rights.* http://www2.ohchr.org/english/law/cescr.htm

United Nations, *Protocol to prevent suppress, and punish trafficking in persons, especially women and children,* supplementing the United Nations *Convention against Transnational Organised Crime* http://www.uncjin.org/Documents/Conventions/dcahistoryl_documents_2/convention_%20traff_eng.pdf

Van Der Maas PJ, Van Delden JJ, Pijnenborg L, Looman CW. Euthanasia and other medical decisions concerning the end of life. *Lancet* 1991 Sep 14; 338(8768):669–74

Wadell, Charles. Clarnette, Roger M. Smith, Michael. Oldham, Lynn. Kellehear, Allan. "Treatment decision-making at the end of life: a survey of Australian doctors' attitudes towards patients' wishes and euthanasia", MJA 165 (540)

White, Thomas Joseph "Jesus' Cry on the Cross and His Beatific Vision" *Nova et Vetera* Vol 5, Issue 3 – Summer 2007 pp, 555–582

Wolf, Susan M., JD, "Gender, Feminism, and Death: Physician-Assisted Suicide and Euthanasia," in Susan M. Woolf Editor *Feminism and Bioethics* Oxford University Press 1996, pp 282–317

Woolf, Susan M. Editor *Feminism and Bioethics* Oxford University Press 1996

World Health Organisation. *Basic documents*. 39th ed. Geneva: WHO, 1992

Index

Abortion
  abortion clinics, 62
  abortion counselling, 62
  child sex abuse, 61
  decriminalisation of, 61
  emergency, 59
  foetal tissue, 58, 62
  nurses duty to assist, 57
  partial birth abortion, 61
  pregnancies to term, 61
  refer for, 58, 63
  termination of pregnancy, 53
Abortion Clinics, 62
Abortion Law Reform Act 2008, 56, 59–60
About Bioethics, Volume One: Philosophical and Theological Approaches
  Tonti-Filippini, Nicholas, 56, 110
Acceptance, 14, 24, 27, 29, 44, 49, 72–73, 97, 130, 168, 179, 185, 194
Act of Euthanasia (May 2002)
  Belgium, 109
  US State of Oregon, 109
Adam and Eve, 160, 170
Address to 1st International Congress on Histopathology of the Nervous System, 87
ADHD, 66
Adrenaline, 76, 174
Advanced care plans
  legal status, 143
Advanced Directive
  Australian jurisdiction, 30, 36, 93
  binding nature, 145
  decisions, 145
  end of life, 198
  failing to comply, 147
  future treatment and care, 143
  homicidal, 138
  legal advice, 93
  living will, 145
  suicidal, 145
  Victorian legislation, 93
Advice, 9, 13, 43, 50–51, 56, 58
Advice on Pregnancy Support and Counselling Services, 58
Agape, 178, 183
Alcohol, 150, 153
Alcoholic, 34, 50
Allocation of Scarce Health Resources
  macro-allocation, 66
  meso-allocation, 66
  micro-allocation, 66
Alter Personality, 155–156
Altruism, 123, 136
Alvarez, ER
  Resuscitation (2006), 77
Alzheimer's disease, 152
Ambulance, 43, 76–77, 79, 164
American Journal of Public Health, 64
American Medical Association, 103, 106
American Psychiatric Association (DSM-IV) Idagnostic and Statiscal Manual, 152
Anaesthesia, 21, 32, 74, 76, 83
Anesthetic, 88, 192
Analysis
  rational, 4
Anathema, 1, 21
Angina, 76, 116
Angiogram, 76
Animal, 82, 162
Anointing of the Sick, 21
Antibiotics, 12, 37, 66, 78–79, 97, 137, 144
a posteriori, 166

207

Index

a priori, 166
Aranda, Sanchia
  Palliative Medicine (2006), 118
Arango
  Schizophrenia Bulletin (2008), 152
Aristotelian
  St. Thomas Aquinas, 166
Arthurs of Nullawil, 75
Ashby, Michael
  Palliative Medicine (2006), 118
Assault
  bodily harm, 32
Assistance, 8, 14, 22, 34, 48, 78, 80, 98,
  103, 108–109, 112, 122, 126, 130,
  139–140, 144, 179, 188
Assisted dying
  Switzerland, 109
Assisted Dying Bill, 104
Assisted Reproductive Technology, 48, 52,
  58, 181
Assisted Suicide, 21, 105, 107–109,
  114, 120
Attitudes
  communitarianism, 121–122
Augustine, St.
  empiricism, 166
  immateriality of the intellect, 166
  Plato, 166
  rationalism, 166
  St. Thomas Aquinas, 166
Australian, 20, 27, 30, 36, 55
Australian Bishops Conference, 58
Australian Constitution, 62
Australian Court, 85
Australian Department of Health and
  Ageing
  National Community Advisory Group
    on Mental Health, 149
Australian Health Ethics Committee, 100
Australian Jurisdiction, 30, 36, 55, 91,
  93–94, 141
Australian Medical Association
  policy on euthanasia, 117
Australian Medical Council (AMC), 47, 54

Australian Medical Practitioner's Board, 47
Australian State of Victoria, 47
Australia's National Statement on Ethical
  Conduct in Human Research, 35,
  52, 58
Authoritarianism, 48
Autism, 152
Autobiographical, 3, 173–174
Autonomy, 2, 21, 33, 48, 56, 69, 97–98,
  105, 121–122, 125–128

Badgery-Parker J., 43
Baume, P., 110
Beatific Vision, 160, 164
Beatitudes
  Christ, 162
  evil, 162
  goodness, 162
  Jesus, 162
  moral values, 162
  suffering, 162
Beeching, Ann
  Nancy, 172
Behaviour, 5, 99, 133
Being a Patient, 159–200
Belgium
  Act of Euthanasia (May 2002), 109
  Death with Dignity Act, 109
Belief
  faith, 5, 25
  religious belief, 46, 55, 98
Believer
  non-believer, 23–24, 179, 182
Berzoff, Joan
  Living with Dying (2004), 18
Best interest, 8–9, 31, 33, 36–39, 46, 50,
  86–87, 91–92, 95, 121
Best Interest Decisions
  substitute judgement, 134
Best Interests principle, 8, 131, 134–136
Bioethics
  Tonti-Filippini, Nicholas, 10
Biographical Life, 99

Blocked airway, 77–79
Bodily integrity, 33, 154
Body
  Christian faith, 23
  human bodiliness, 24
  integration of, 23
Bolam Principle, 41
Bolam test, 41
Bolam v Friern Hospital Management
    Committee (1957), 41
Brain damage, 43, 75, 82
Bride
  Church, 169
Bridegroom
  Christ, 169
British Medical Association, 103–104
Brother, 43, 82, 99, 137
Burden
  of illness, 65
  of suffering, 65
  to others, 98, 112, 114, 118, 178, 180
Burdensome
  burdensome life, 26, 107, 110,
      112, 117
  overly burdensome, 7–8, 22, 78–79, 81,
      86, 90
  treatment, 74, 78, 97, 199
Burden to others, 98, 112, 114, 118,
    178–182

Canadian Medical Association, 103, 105
Cancer
  patients, 77, 113
Capital Punishment, 10
Cardiac Arrest, 77
Cardinal
  John Henry Newman, 5
Care
  burden of, 47
  duty of, 47
  extraordinary means, 73
  institutional care, 67, 70
  intensive, 8, 13, 21–22, 77, 174, 188

medical care, 19, 50, 52, 82, 103, 199
  negligence, 32, 37
  of the dying, 7, 71, 77, 81, 117, 144
  ordinary means, 73
  palliative, 18, 20, 86–89
  psychological, 47
  reasonable, 29, 33, 41, 72, 86, 97
Care of the Dying and Proportionate
    Means, 71–77, 81, 144
Care until the End, 71–120
Caring Relationships, 11–70
Caritas in Veritate, 64–65
Catchlove, Dr Barry
  Royal Children's Hospital,
      Melbourne, 177
Catechism of the Catholic
    Church, 72, 163
Catholic
  Church, 4, 96, 199
  faith, 5, 167
  Pope, 2, 4
  Vatican, 161
Catholic Bishops, 58
Catholic Church, 4, 96, 199
Catholic Health Australia
  Code of Ethic Standards, 53
Catholic tradition, 25, 72, 139, 143, 185
Celibate
  union with God, 168
Celso
  Schizophrenia Bulletin (2008), 152
Cerebral haemorrhage, 85
Charity
  communion, 65
  forgiving, 65
  God's love in human relationships, 65
  gratuitiousness, 65
  justice, 65
  mercy, 65
  salvific value, 65
  transcends justice, 65
Charter of Human Rights and
    Responsibilities Bill, 60
Cheesman, Denis

diabetes, 176
Friedrich's Ataxia, 176
neediness, 177
to be more human, 177
Chemotherapy, 75, 184
Childbirth
  empathy, 189
  pain, 187–188
Christ
  bridegroom, 169
  Christ as god, 165
  Cross, 169
  death and resurrection, 161
  death of, 162, 182
  father, 163–164
  healed both physically and spiritually, 160
  Jesus, 160
  life, 160
  mystery, 161
  redeemer, 159
  resurrection, 159
  sacrifice, 71
  significance for us, 159
  sin, 159
  submission to the father, 71
  suffering, 161
Christian
  Christian physician, 160
  embodied, 161
  faith, 160
  human love, 160
Christian Bioethics, 74, 176
Christianity
  God, 183
  Judaism, 183
  love of neighbour, 183
  virtues, 182
Christians
  faith, 4–6
  Ministry, 159
  new beginning, 71
  responsible stewards, 139
Christological, 24, 161

Chronic Illness
  burden of chronically ill, 18
  provision of Palliative Care, 112
Chronic Pain, 19, 112–113, 187–189
Church
  bride, 169
  Catholic, 4, 72, 96, 199
  Christ, 170
  communitarianism, 121–122
Clark, Peter, 74
Clarnette, Roger M.
  MJA 165 (540), 110
Clinical decisions, 44, 154
Clinicians, 3, 48
Clone, 11
Code of ethics, 57–58
Coercion
  freedom from, 32
Cognitively impaired, 32, 133
Cole, JA, 43
Coma
  quality of life, 67, 100
  state of consciousness, 83
  unresponsive, 82
Comedy, 172
Common Good, 72
Commonwealth, 62, 112, 119
Communication
  effective, 46
Communion, 65, 71, 127, 160, 168, 170–171, 173, 175, 185
Communion of persons, 170, 173
Communio Personarum (Communion of persons), 166
Communitarian attitudes, 122
Communitarianism
  Church, 121
  individualism, 121–122, 127, 136, 200
Community
  attitudes, 20
  communio personarum, 166
  equal basis, 128
  family, 121, 130
  individualism, 127

Index   211

love, 127
of persons, 166
participation, 128, 130
Companionship, 173
Competence, 11, 32–35
Competitiveness, 20
Concepts, 2, 6, 17, 46
Conduct
   immoral, 53, 153
   unethical, 53
Confidentiality, 20, 157
Conflict of interest, 137
Conscience
   contrary to, 53
   freedom of, 48, 55, 145
   professional, 47–63
Conscientious objection, 48–49, 51–59
Consciousness, 83, 99–100
Consensus, 2–3, 6, 61
Consent
   informed, 8, 14–15, 20, 29, 33, 145, 200
Consequentialism, 181
Contract, 32, 38
Convention on the Rights of People with Disabilities, 128, 130
Cooper, Adam, 10
Cooperation
   in an act, 53
   with evil, 10
Cosmetic surgery, 38, 54, 68, 125
Counselling, 27, 58, 61–62, 87
Court
   Australian, 85
   Supreme, 85
Coyte, Anthony, 10
Creator, 4, 22, 185–186
Crimes Act, 30–31, 61, 94, 123, 131
Criminal law, 94, 107, 131
Critical interests, 36, 150
Cross of Christ, 163, 169, 173
Crown Prosecution Service, 108–109
Cult of the Body, 72
Cultural Influences, 4
Culture, 1, 3–4, 8, 12, 19, 21, 26, 51,
   139–140, 181

D'Arcy, Archbishop Eric, 11
Daughter, 43, 82, 99, 157, 171, 184
Death
   accepting, 139
   by active intervention, 97
   by neglect, 97
   cause, 73, 95
   farewell, 165
   imminent death, 94, 186
   prolongation of life, 97
Deception, 45, 155
Decision
   altruistic, 123
   best interest, 134
   clinical, 44, 154
   exploitative, 126
   financial, 122–123, 147
   harmful, 126
Decision maker, 32, 131–132
Decision making, 20, 33–34, 50, 58, 62,
   110, 121–122, 124, 127, 134
Decision-making capacity
   impaired, 62, 124, 126–127
Defendant, 41, 43
Defibrillation, 77, 144
Dehydration
   cognitive effects, 88–89
   headaches, 88
   muscle cramps, 88
   pain, 88
   renal failure, 88
Dementia, 33–34, 70, 80–81, 122, 130,
   137–138
Democracy, 99
Depression, 19, 78, 89, 149–150,
   152, 179
De Profundis
   Psalm 130, 167, 185
Despair, 162–163, 180–181, 194
De Trinitate, 166
De Vitoria, Francisco
   Relectiones Theologicae, 74

Diabetes, 176
Diagnosis, 13, 16, 39–40, 44–45, 49, 66, 84, 149, 152–155, 195–196
Dialogue with Trypho, 163
Dialysis, 9, 64, 76, 144, 181, 197
Dignity
  autonomy, 126–128
  equal rights, 125
  human dignity, 3, 82, 125, 127, 132
  inalienable rights, 129, 132
  inherent dignity, 11, 124–125, 127–130
  intrinsic value, 82
  inviolability, 27, 99, 125, 131–132
  Pope John Paul II, 96
  Prostitution, 125–126
  Representation, 124–126
Directive
  failing to comply, 147
  representative, 147
Disability
  and chronic illness, 18, 26, 173
  community, 178
  Hayes, Susan, 175
  mystery of disability, 175
Disabled, 28, 43, 67, 82, 102, 105, 110–111, 116, 126, 153, 175–176
Disease
  advanced disease, 113, 118
  causes of, 28
  prevention of, 66
Distribution of Goods, 64
Divine
  divine image, 24, 161, 166
  divine love, 6, 170, 178, 187, 190, 195
  God, 22
  union with God, 168
Divine image, 24, 161, 166
Dlugoborski
  Auschwitz, 1940–1945, 88
Doctor
  competence, 32
  ethical credibility, 110
  medical practitioner, 47, 57
  protection of, 56
  skills, 11, 41, 49
Doctrine
  of creation, 23
  of incarnation, 23
Dogma, 15, 23, 29
Donation, 10, 23, 52, 58
Double effect reasoning, 28
Down Syndrome
  infertile, 176
Drug(s)
  addicted, 34
Drugs, Poisons and Controlled Substances Act 1981, 57, 137
Drug Tolerance, 19
Dualism
  unity, 23, 99
Duty of Care
  obligation to Provide Care, 87
Dworkin, Ronald
  narrative wreck, 178
Dying
  live more fully with, 112
  process, 18, 20–21, 25, 71, 100, 102, 106, 112, 139, 198
Dykxhoorn, Hermina
  euthanasiam, 108

Earthly pilgrimage, 71
Economic Rationalism, 84
Effects of Sin, 159–160, 189
Eiser, Arnold R., 145
Elderly, 14, 28, 69–70, 78, 98, 101–102, 105–107, 114, 144, 182
Electro-convulsive therapy, 155
Elliott, Bishop Peter, 10
Elwyn, Glyn
  Palliative Medicine (2005), 113, 118
Embryo
  implantation, 53
Emergency, 30, 32, 57, 59, 93
Emergency Assistance, 22
Emergency Treatment, 30, 87, 93
Emotions, 18, 184, 191
Empathy

community, 168
dying, 118
Edith Stein, 159, 191
illness, 191
love, 192
suffering, 192
support of others, 72, 118
unity, 168
Empiricism, 166
Employment, 19, 63, 95, 178
Encyclical
  Caritas in Veritate, 64
End of life, 84, 92, 102, 106, 110, 174, 178–179, 181, 198–199
End of life decisions, 139
Enduring attorney, 146
Enduring guardian, 146
Enduring Power of Attorney, 36, 86, 144
Environment
  sustainability, 26
Epilepsy, 43
Eros, 178, 183
Eternal life, 160
Ethical concernsEthical considerationsEthical Guidelines, 20, 47, 52, 176
Ethical Guidelines for the Care of People in Post Coma Unresponsiveness (Vegative State) or a Minimally Responsive State, 100
Ethical Guidelines on the Use of Assisted Reproductive Technology in Clinical Practice and Research, 52
Ethical objection, 55
Ethics
  code of, 53, 57–58, 199
  ideal, 29
  standards, 50, 53, 55–56
  utilitarianism ethics, 67
Ethics, Creation and Environment, 4, 10
Eucharist, 21
Euthanasia
  action, 93, 96
  active, 95
  by sedation, 109
  Catholic Church on, 96
  drug overdose, 96
  infants with abnormalities, 110
  intervention, 94
  involuntarym, 96
  killing, 96
  law, 96
  legalized, 112, 119
  legalising of, 99, 107
  legislation, 112–120
  medically-assisted dying, 102–103
  mercy-killing, 107
  Netherlands, 108
  non-voluntary, 96
  omission, 96
  passive, 95–96
  psychiatrist, 115
  psychosocial concerns, 113
  violation of the law of god, 96
  voluntary, 95
  women, 114
Euthanasia Legislation
  unbearable pain, 107, 117
Evangelium Vitae, 96, 162
Evil
  goodness, 162
  moral values, 162
  pinckaers, servais, 162
  problem of evil, 162
  suffering, 162
Evolutionary Process, 26
Examination
  physical, 15
Existence
  purpose of, 61
Existential
  suffering, 65, 178–180
Existential Pain
  loneliness, 117
  self worth, 117
Existential Suffering, 65, 178–180
Exploitation, 129, 131
Extraordinary means, 73

Faculties
  lower functions, 27
  mental, 27
  mental functions, 27
  physical, 27
  spiritual, 28
Fagerlin, Angela
  Enough: The Failure of the Living Will
    (2004), 145–146
Faith
  Adam and Eve, 160, 170
  beatific vision, 160
  Christian, 23
  embodied, 161
  eternal life, 160
  fall of man, 160
  human love, 160
  immortal soul, 160
  mystery, 161
  original sin, 160
  prayer, 163–165
  prophetic fulfillment, 163
  sanctification, 160
  sin and suffering, 160
Faith experience, 174
Fallen nature, 71
Fall of Man, 160
Families, 19, 46–47, 70, 111, 115, 117,
    140, 157, 166, 176
Families and Confidentiality, 157
Fatal treatment, 96, 100
Father, 48, 69, 71, 81–82, 98–99, 163–166,
    170, 173, 183–186, 194
Feeding
  loss of, 83
  spoon-feeding, 84
  tube feeding, 74–84
Feminism and Bioethics (1996), 114
Fertility decline
  aged people, 70
Fiduciary Model, 39
Filippini, Contessa (Nancy), 172

Financial decisions, 122–123, 147
Fleming, John
  *Seeking an Australian Consensus on
    Abortion and Sex Education*
    (2007), 27
Foetal Tissue, 58, 62
Foetus, 27, 49, 53, 58, 61–62
  legal status, 61
Food
  refusal of, 84
Force-feeding, 88
Form and matter
  St. Thomas Aquinas, 166–167
Fragility, 26, 107–120
Freedom
  belief, 33, 48, 60, 63, 145
  conscience, 33, 48, 54–55, 60,
    63, 145
  of thought, 33, 48, 54–55, 60,
    63, 145
Free Market, 16, 38, 41
Freewill, 71, 97, 161, 187, 189
Friendship
  friendship with God, 176
Fruitful love, 170
Future Care, 138–141, 198
Future Care Plan Statement, 140

Gaudium et Spes, 24, 161
Gay unions, 118
Gender, 12–13, 53, 67
Genesis, 189
Gesthsemane, 71, 139, 193–194
Gift, 72, 139, 165, 169–173, 183
Gift of Self, 4, 169, 172
God
  Christ, 161, 163, 165, 169
  divine, 166
  Father, 163
  friendship with god, 176
  grace, 21–22
  Holy Spirit, 171
  image of, 23–24, 161, 173

Index

intimacy of God, 170
Jesus, 160, 163
  loving, 24
  omniscient, 165
  praise for God, 163
  presence, 21, 185
  Psalm, 163
  relationship to, 165
  separation from, 160
  sin, 160
  works of God, 161, 191
God's love
  agape, 178, 183
  analogy, 183
  charity, 185
  eros, 178, 183
  justice, 200
  love of one's spouse, 171
  mercy, 65
  witness to, 160, 194
God's will, 139, 161
Good
  perfect, 23
Good life, 97
Good Medical Practice: A Code of Conduct for Australia's Doctors, 47, 49, 51
Government pharmaceutical subsidies, 113
Grace, 21–22, 170–171, 185–186, 200
Grandparents, 70
Greece, 20
Greg, 76
Guardian, 35–36, 86, 126, 146
Guardianship, 121, 124
Guardianship and Administration Act 2000 (Qld), 93, 122, 134
Guardianship law, 121, 124
Gynaecology, 63

Habitat, 26
Haemodialysis, 116, 199
Hanson, RPC
  Justin Martyr's Dialogue with Trypho

(1963), 163
Happiness, 18, 24, 66, 133, 161–162, 172
Harman, Fr Francis, 193
Hayes, R.
  Mental Retardation (1982), 175
HAYES, Susan C.
  Mental Retardation (1982), 175
Health
  health care, 7, 11–12, 19, 25, 28
  health resources, 63
  mental health, 17, 25, 122, 133–134
  reproductive health, 17
  spiritual health, 17
  well-being, 65–66
Health Care
  causes of disease, 28
  ethics, 7
  longevity, 63
  prevent disease, 28
  rationing of, 66, 69
  standards, 63–64
  utilitarian, 67
Health Insurance companies, 69
Health Resources
  allocation of, 63, 66
Health Services
  care, 51
  duty, 57
  empathy, 65
  love, 65
Heart surgery, 76
Heart transplant, 76
Hippocrates, 103
Hippocratic Oath, 29, 103
Hippocratic Tradition, 50
Hodgkin's disease, 68
Holy Spirit, 171, 186
Homicidal, 92, 135, 138
Hope(s)
  resurrection, 28
Hospital, 7, 11–12, 16–17, 33, 43, 45, 57, 74, 77, 86–87, 93–94, 111, 137, 144, 151, 164, 174, 181, 184–185, 196

Hudson Peter
  Palliative Medicine (2006), 118
Hudson, Rosalie
  Palliative Medicine (2006), 118
Hulls, Rob
  Charter of Human Rights and
    Responsibilities Bill 2006, 60
Human
  neediness, 177
Human Being
  characteristic of, 162
  divine image and likeness, 166
  Imago Dei, 22–28
  Trinitarian anthropology, 165
Human Body
  Imago Dei, 24
Human Condition
  death, 71, 97, 139
  sin, 71, 139
Human Dignity
  violation of, 132
Human Family, 82, 99, 106, 125, 129,
    131–132, 173, 175, 178
Human genome, 175
Human Good, 1–2, 38
Human identity, 25, 127
Human life
  inviolability of, 27, 99
  sanctity of, 98–99
Human love
  human suffering, 171
  Judaeo-Christian, 183
  love of God, 183
Human Person
  bodily dimension, 161
  christological, 161
  divine image, 161
  spiritual, 161
  Trinitarian mystery, 166
Human Research Ethics Committee, 9
Human Rights
  protecting human rights, 3
Human Rights Committee (UN), 119
Human will

Hunger-striking, 101
Hunter, Toby, 10
Hurst, Samia A.
  BMJ 2003, 109
Hydration
  refusal of, 84

Illicit drugs, 137
Illness
  acute, 174
  chronic, 18, 26, 67, 115, 117, 173, 179
  degenerative, 8, 110, 142, 144, 174
  mental, 8, 69, 89, 108, 122, 149
  psychiatric, 86, 89, 95
  terminal illness, 39, 85, 105, 110, 116,
    141, 199
Image and Likeness of God
  communion, 71, 175
  freewill, 189
Imago Dei
  human bodiliness, 24, 161
Immateriality of the intellect, 166
Immortality, 24
Impairments, 33, 35, 81, 122, 128, 132,
    149, 151, 175, 199
Incarnation, 23
Incontinence, 70
Individual, 1, 3, 11, 15–16, 20, 23, 25, 34,
    65, 68–69, 103–104, 111, 114, 123,
    125–130, 133, 136, 149–150, 155,
    174, 179, 183, 185
Individualism, 1, 8, 121–122, 127–129,
    136, 181, 200
Industrial Revolution, 11
Industry, 7, 11
Infection
  lung, 12, 14, 21
  respiratory, 8, 12, 16
Infertile, 176
Infertility treatment, 68
Information
  blocking of, 46
  sharing, 40
Informed Consent, 8, 14–15, 20, 29, 33,

Index

145, 200
Institutional Care, 67, 70
Instrumental Value
  intrinsic value, 82
Integration of the body, 23
Intellect
  Augustine, St., 166
Intensive Care, 8, 13, 21–22, 77, 174, 188
International Congress on Life
  Sustaining Treatment and the
  Vegetative State, 81
International Covenants
  Civil and Political Rights, 54, 62,
  119, 129
  Economical, Social and Cultural
  Rights, 129
International Human Rights instruments,
  119, 124–125, 132
International Human Rights law, 99
International Theological Commission
  *Communion and Stewardship: Human
  Persons Created in the Image of God*
  (2002), 23, 161
Interpreter, 40
Intervention
  active, 97
  assent to, 28
  non-therapeutic, 50
  patient, 50
  prevent suicide, 87
Intrinsic, 23, 82, 105–106
Intubation, 21, 76, 78–79, 144
Inviolability of human life, 27, 99
Involuntary
  patient, 9
Irenaeus, St., 163
Ischaemic Heart Disease, 75–76, 80–81,
  110, 198
Islamic, 19
Isolation of the patient, 45, 65
Italian, 19, 172

Jerome, St., 163
Jesus
  as friend, 173
  as lover, 173
  as man, 164
  as teacher, 173
  beatitudes, 162
  Christ, 186
  Cross, 171
  Cry, 171
  final cry, 173
  healed both physically and spiritually, 160
  humanity, 160
  loss of self, 164
  prayer, 163–165
  prophetic fulfillment, 163
  relationship to the Father, 164
  solidarity with sinners, 163
  St. Justin the Martyr, 163
  union, 168–169
Jesus' cry
  comfort from, 164
  extreme suffering, 163–164
  final cry, 163–164
  mystery, 165–166
  solitariness of suffering, 165
  St. Justin of Martyr, 163
  St. Thomas, 164
  Suffering, 162–164
John Paul II Institute for Marriage
  and Family, 10
Johns, Brian
  Down Syndrome, 175–176
Joy, 10, 22, 25, 162, 168, 173, 175, 187,
  200
Judaism, 183
Judgement
  evidence-based, 50
  mistaken, 33
  professional, 50
  unethical, 50
Justice
  distribution of goods, 64
  liberty, 64
Justin the Martyr, St., 163
Just War Theory, 10

Kahn, René
   Schizophrenia Bulletin (2008), 152
Kant, Immanuel, 98
Karlo, 45
Kellehear, Allan
   MJA 165 (540), 110
Kelly, Brian
   Palliative Medicine (2006), 118
Kerridge, Ian
   MJA Vol 190, 48
Killing
   by omission, 96
   euthanasia, 96
   mercy-killing, 107
   physician-assisted suicide, 69, 98, 102–107
Kilner, John
   Who Lives? Who Dies? (1984), 66
Kinney, Graham, 137
Kirby, P., 43, 133
Kissane, David W.
   Seven deaths in Darwin: case studies (1998), 115, 119
Klein, Rudolf
   Lessons for (and From) America (2003), 64
Komesaroff, Paul A.
   MJA Vol 190, 48
Kommesaroff, Paul, 48
Kristjanson, Linda J.
   Palliative Medicine (2006), 118

Lancet (1991), 110, 115, 119
Lateran University (Rome), 111
Law
   Australian jurisdiction, 30, 36, 55, 91, 93–94, 141
   criminal law statutes, 107
   equal opportunity, 48
   Federal, 48
   moral, 89
   morality, 27, 89
   reform, 6
   State, 48
   Territory, 48
   Victorian, 8, 62
Legal medications, 109
Legal Rights, 61, 78
Legislation
   ideology, 116
Lethargy, 88
Liberalism, 127
Life
   biographical, 99
   biological, 99
   eternal life, 160
   hopes and goals, 140
   journey, 25
   last phase of, 71
   life as a gift, 139
   mystery, 139
   next life, 20
   person, 100
   physical, 99
   preserving life, 28, 74
   prolonging of, 78, 86, 96, 109
   sacredness of, 98
   value, 100
Life-prolonging treatment, 86, 96, 109
Life-Sustaining Treatments and Vegetative State, 81
Life-threatening situation, 28, 144
Listening
   open-ended questions, 46
Living, 18–19, 26, 41, 73, 107–110
Living Will
   advanced directives, 8, 92–93, 138, 143–146
Loneliness
   divine love, 6, 170, 178, 187, 190, 195
   existential suffering, 178–180
   suffering, 175–178
Longevity, 63
Looman CW
   Lancet 1991, 110
Lord Joel Joffe, 104
Loss of control, 19

Index

Love
  communio personarum, 166
  divine love, 6, 170, 178, 187, 190, 195
  fruitful love, 170
  god's love, 22–24, 65, 160, 170, 176, 183, 185, 187, 193, 195
  love of god, 26, 171, 183, 194
  love of neighbour, 73, 183
  marital love, 6, 169, 183
  reciprocity, 20, 182–183
  spousal love, 170, 187
Love of God, 26, 171, 183, 194
Love of neighbour, 73, 183
Love of self, 73
Lumen Gentium, 170
Lung infection, 12, 14, 21

MacIntyre, Alasdair
  The Tasks of Philosophy: Selected Essays (2006), 4
Macro-allocation
  queuing, 66
Mahoney JA, 43
Mak, Yvonne Yi Wood
  Palliative Medicine (2005), 113
Malice, 34, 37
Mannix College, 176
Marital love
  Paul VI, 169
  John Paul II, 169
  gift of self, 169
  empathy, 169
  communion of persons, 170
Marriage
  Christian marriage, 23
  couple, 170
  marital love, 169
  marriage relationship, 169
  sacrament of marriage, 170–172
Marriage relationship
  covenant, 169
  holiness, 169
  love, 169

Married person, 168, 173
Mass
  Catholic, 167
  Christ, 167
  cross, 169
  prayer, 165
Mattson MP 2005
  Annual Review of Nutrition Volume 25, 88
Maturity, 35
Mauron, Alex
  BMJ 2003, 109
McNair, Justice, 41
Medical Care
  ethos of medical care, 103
Medical Doctor, 22
Medical Journal of Australia, 93, 137
Medically-assisted dying, 102–103
Medical Practitioner, 42, 56–57, 104, 110, 115, 142, 146
Medical Profession, 103
Medical Treatment
  decision, 144
  enduring power of attorney, 36, 86, 144
Medications
  lethal medications, 109
  self-administration of, 109
Medicine
  alternative medicine, 50
  ethos of medicine, 102
  psychiatric medicine, 154
  truth-telling, 154
Memory, 34, 152–154, 196
Mental Competence, 90
Mental function, 27
Mental Health, 17, 25, 122, 133–134, 149, 154, 157
Mental Illness
  Alzheimer's disease, 152
  American Psychiatric Association (DSM-IV) Idagnostic and Statiscal Manual, 152
  anxiety, 150
  Australian Department of Health and

Ageing, 149
bipolar, 150
classifying, 151–152
critical interests, 150
delusions, 150
depression, 150
ethics and mental illness, 149
hallucinations, 150
National Community Advisory Group on Mental Health, 149
neurosis, 150
obsessive compulsive disorder, 150
phobia, 150
post-trauma syndromes, 150
psychosis, 150
psychosomatic disorders, 150
psychotic disorders, 150
Schizophrenia, 150–152
self-harm, 157
WHO International Classifications of Diseases (ICD-10), 152
Mercy, 65
Mercy-killing
  Belgium, 109
  Netherlands, 107
  prohibition of, 110
  US State of Oregon, 109
Meso-allocation, 66–67
Metaphysical, 23, 61
Micro-allocation, 66–67
Middle Ages, 26
Mind, 18, 27–28, 78, 85–87, 90, 92, 115, 138, 146, 157, 164, 172, 181, 188, 195
Monash University, 111, 176–177
Moral
  acts, 4
  dilemma, 26
Morality, 27, 72, 89
Morally neutral act, 53
Morphine, 164
Mother, 43, 48, 61, 70, 82, 99, 151, 157, 182–186
Motherhood, 10, 27, 166

Multiple Sclerosis, 14, 144
Multugera of Jagara, 75
Munsell MF
  Resuscitation (2006), 77

Nancy
  An Autobiography of Filippini, Contessa (1988), 172
Narrative Wreck
  Dworkin, Ronald, 178
Naso-gastric Tube, 79–81
National Health and Medical Research Council (NHMRC), 2, 35–36, 40, 46, 52, 58, 100, 111, 123, 150, 176
National Statement on Ethical Conduct in Human Research, 35, 52, 58
Natural world, 26
Nature
  fallen, 71
Nausea, 14
Neediness, 177
Needs
  communitarian, 8
Negligence, 32, 37, 41
Netherlands, 101, 107–108, 114, 119–120
Neuberger, Julia
  BMJ. 2003, 18
Newman, John Henry
  doctrinal development, 5–6
New Zealand Bill of Rights, 85
New Zealand Medical Association, 103, 105
Next of kin, 36, 79, 86, 137, 141, 198–199
Nitschke, Philip
  Seven deaths in Darwin: case studies (1998), 115, 119
Northern Territory Rights of the Terminally Ill Act, 115, 119
Not For Resuscitation, 7, 76–79
Not For Resuscitation Orders
  next of kin, 79
Nova et Vetera, 2, 107
Nurse

Index

duty to assist, 57, 59
late term abortion, 59
Nursing Home, 11, 37, 77
Nutrition
　artificial, 85
Nutrition and Hydration
　refusal of, 84–85

Obligation to Provide Care, 32, 39,
　87–88, 90
Obstetric care, 68
O'Connor, Margaret
　Christian Bioethics (2006), 118
OECD Health Data 2006, 63
Oldham, Lynn
　MJA 165 (540)
O'Malley E., 110
Ophthalmia, 42
Order of Malta, 180
OrganOrgan and Tissue Donation after
　Death, for Transplantation, 52
Organ Donation, 23, 58
Organ Donor, 123
Organ Failure, 88
Organisation for Economic Co-operation
　and Development, 63
Original Sin
　Fall of Man, 160
O'Rourke, Kevin
　Christian Bioethics (2006), 176
O'Shea, Gerard, 10
Ouellet, Marc
　Trinitarian Anthropology of the Family,
　166, 171
Overdose, 96–97, 137

Paediatric Neurologist, 43
Page, Margaret, 85
Pain
　acute, 19
　adrenaline, 76, 164
　childbirth, 187
　chronic, 19, 112–113, 187–189

existential pain, 117
morphine, 164
relief, 62, 86, 89, 113, 118, 188
self-hypnotherapy, 188
unbearable, 107, 117
Pain relief, 62, 86, 89, 113, 118, 188
Palliative Care
　pain, 118
　palliative care facilities, 113
　spiritual elements, 118
　suffering, 118
　suicidal project, 87, 89
Paralysis
　Pope John Paul II, 193
Parenthood, 9
Parenting, 48, 173, 175
Parents
　honour of, 183
Parkinson's Disease, 80
Partial Birth Abortion, 61
Participation
　barriers, 128
Passions, 18
Passive, 19, 95–96, 191
Paternalism
　strong paternalism, 33
　weak paternalism, 33
Patient(s)
　being a patient, 159
　future care planning, 140–141
　patient centeredness, 49
　persuation of, 88, 95
　restraining, 88
　rights of, 91
　vulnerability of, 55
Patient-centeredness, 49
Patient-doctor relationships, 102
Patterson, Colin, 10
Peace, 21, 44, 77, 129, 162, 186, 193
Percutaneous Endoscopic Gastroscopy,
　79, 88
Permission
　direct, 87

explicit, 87
implicit, 87
indirect, 87
Person
   human, 1–2, 18, 21, 23–25, 27, 96, 129, 161, 166
   married person, 168, 173
Personality
   anti-social, 156
Pharmacist, 56–57
Philosopher
   respect, 175
Phyllis, Silverman
   Living with Dying (2004), 18
Physical, 15, 18, 23, 27–28, 61, 65, 72, 88–89, 99, 108, 113, 118, 122, 126, 128, 152–153, 160, 186, 188, 191, 193, 198
Physician
   Christian physician, 160
Physician-Assisted Suicide
   legalising of physician-assisted suicide, 106
   statement on physician assisted suicide, 103
Pijnenborg L
   Lancet 1991, 110
Pinckaers, Servais
   The Sources of Christian Ethics (1995), 162
Piper, Franciszek
   uschwitz, 1940–1945, 88
Placebos
   dummy treatment, 155
Planet, 25
Planning
   future care, 138–139
Planning future care
   desirability of future care planning, 140
   future care, 198
Plato, 166
Pneumonia, 80, 85, 100, 174
Policy(ies)
   liberal policies, 118
   public, 6, 121

reproductive technology, 118
social policies, 118
Politicians, 115
Pope Benedict XVI
   Caritas in Veritate (2009), 64
   Ratzinger, Joseph, 4
Pope John Paul II
   Catholic Church, 96
   celibate, 168
   Dives in Misericordia, 162
   Evangelium Vitae, 162
   Familiaris Consortio, 24
   Gaudium et Spes, 24, 161
   Letter to Families, 166, 169
   marriage, 10, 166
   paralysis, 193
   relationship, 168
   Trinitarian anthropology, 159, 165, 167
   Vatican, 24
   vocation, 168
Pope Paul VI
   couples, 169
   relationship, 169
Pope Pius XII, 4, 87–88, 90, 187
Population
   age, 69
   declining fertility, 69
   economic circumstances, 70
Power of Attorney, 36, 86, 90, 144, 147
Prayer, 163–165, 171, 185–186, 194, 197
Pregnant, 57, 59, 61
Preserving life
   disproportionate, 97
   extraordinary, 74, 97
   ordinary, 74
   proportionate, 97
Prevent suicide
   Intervention, 94
   use of reasonable force, 94
Priest
   Minister, 59
Primum non nocere (first do no harm), 155

Index

Principle of Totality, 27–28
Principles of Healthcare, 25–28
Prison Reform Society, 76
Professional Conscience, 47–63
Prognosis, 36, 38–40, 44–45, 47, 113, 142, 176
Proportionate Means, 71–77
Prostitution
  sex worker, 132
Protection of individual life, liberty and security, 125
Psalm
  God, 163
  prayer, 197
Psychiatric illnesses, 86
Psychiatric medicine, 154
Psychiatric Treatments
  alter personality, 155
  electro-convulsive therapy, 155
  placebos, 155
  psychotherapy, 155
  ranking, 155
Psychiatry
  criminality, 156
  misused, 131
  social uses of psychiatry, 156–157
Psychic reality, 168
Psychological care, 47
Psychologists, 56–58
Psychometric index of quality, 68
Psychosomatic functioning, 65
Public Advocate, 137
Public authority (guardianship), 90

Quadriplegic
  Cheesman, Denis, 176
Quality Adjusted Life Years
  Quality of Life, 67
Quality of Life, 67, 100, 104, 111, 177
Queensland Guardianship and Administration Act 2000, 93, 122, 134
Queensland Powers of Attorney Act 1998, 93

Radiotherapy, 75
Ranking Psychiatric Treatments, 155
Rape, 132
Rationalism, 84, 166
Ratzinger, Joseph, 4
Reason
  contrary to, 24
Reasonable Care, 29, 33, 41, 72, 86, 97
Reasonable force to Prevent Suicide, 30, 94–95, 131
Reconciliation, 21
Referrals, 52–53, 125
Refusal of Food and Water
  hunger-striking, 101
  obligation to provide care, 87–88
  palliative care, 88–89
  secondary psychiatric illness, 89–90
Refusal to eat, 86
Registration, 47
Reisfield GM
  Resuscitation (2006), 77
Relationship(s)
  dependence, 126–128
  trinity, 165
  with creator, 22
  with God, 160, 170
  with other persons, 21
Relectiones Theologicae, 74
Religious, 2, 52, 54–55
Religious belief
  prayer, 55
Renal Disease, 12, 14
Representation
  altruism, 123
  Disability Act (2006, Victoria), 122
  Guardianship and Administration Act 1985 (Victoria)
  guardianship law, 124
  Medical Treatment Act (1998, Victoria), 122, 146
  Mental Health Act (1986, Victoria), 122
Representation and Disability, 121–147
Representative
  appointing, 142

appointment of, 137
best interest, 147
elders, 143
evaluating medical decisions, 44
guiding, 143
guiding one's representative, 141
homicidal, 92
Ministers, 143
pastoral carers, 143
substituted consent, 138
Represented Decisions
mental competence, 90
power of attorney, 90
public authority (guardianship), 90
Reproductive Health, 17
Reproductive technology, 48, 52, 58, 118, 181
Resources, 26, 60, 63–70
Respect
for truth, 5
Respiratory failure, 78
Respiratory infection, 8, 12
Resurrection
Christ, 161
hope, 28
Resuscitation
cardiac massage, 78
defribillation, 78
futile, 78
intubation, 78
not for resuscitation orders, 76–79
overly burdensome, 78
para-medical, 79
Revelation
Beatific vision, 160
eternal life, 160
Imago Dei, 159
sanctification, 160
Right(s)
inalienable and equality of rights, 125
inherent human dignity, 125
International Human Rights instruments, 125
of the patient, 91
to freedom of conscience, 145
to freedom of religion, 60
to freedom of thought, 33, 54–55, 60, 62–63
to say no, 94
Right to life, 60–61, 99, 119, 132
Rogers Principle, 43
Rogers v. Whitaker, 42
Romans, 81
Rossiter case, 85, 90
Rossiter, Christian, 85, 90
Rowland, Tracey, 1, 10
Royal Australian College of Nursing, 58
Royal Childen's Hospital, Melbourne, 177
Royal Medical Society, 107

Sacramental Grace, 170–171
Sacrament of marriage
unity, 170, 172
Sacrifice
of Christ, 71
Salvation
of our souls, 72
Sanctification, 160
Sanctity of human life, 98
Saracci, Rodolfo, 18
Saviour, 22
Savulescu, Julian, 49
Scarman, Lord, 41
Schizophrenia, 150–152, 174
Schneider, Carl E.
Enough: The Failure of the Living Will (2004), 145–146
Schofield, Penelope
Palliative Medicine (2006), 118
Science
human genome, 175
modern science, 175
philosopher, 47
Secondary Psychiatric Illness, 86, 89–90, 95
Second Vatican Council
Gaudium et Spes, 24, 161

Secular
  society, 6
Self Image, 19, 196
Self worth, 117, 178
Service, 7, 11–29
Sexual intimacy
  sexually abused, 152
Sexuality, 10
Sexually abused, 152
Sexual orientation, 153
Sexual preference, 153
Sexual promiscuity, 153
Sex worker
  prostitution, 125
Sidaway v. Governors of Bethlem Royal Hospital, 41
Side effects, 14–15, 28, 39–40, 89, 140, 155, 184, 198
Sin
  Adam and Eve, 160
  and suffering, 160
  effects of, 159–160, 189
  Fall of man, 160
  fallen nature, 71
  original sin, 160
  power of, 159
Sister, 82, 99, 185
Smart, JJC
  An Outline of a System of Utilitarianism Ethics, 67
Smith, Michael
  MJA 165 (540), 110
Social Uses of Psychiatry, 156–157
Society
  Convention on the Rights of Persons with Disabilities, 128
  inclusion in, 130
Solidarity, 73, 115, 163
Solzhenitsyn, Alexander
  totalitarian regimes, 156
Soul
  immateriality of the intellect, 166
  immortal soul, 23, 160
Species

  loss of, 26
Spiritual, 23–24, 28, 55, 118, 154, 161, 163, 173
Spiritual Health, 17
Sports, 72
Spousal love, 170, 187
Spouse
  intimacy of god, 170
  marriage, 171
  spousal love, 170, 187
  suffering of a spouse, 170
  trinity, 169
Starvation
  dehydration, 88
  distress, 88
  lethargy, 88
  organ failure, 88
  pain, 88
State of Consciousness
  coma, 82
Status
  protected, 110, 114
Stein, Edith (Teresa Benedicta, St.)
  empathy, 159
  psychic reality, 168
  On the Problem of Empathy (1964), 168, 191
Stem cells, 58
Stewards, 26, 73, 139
Stewardship
  responsible stewardship, 25
Street, Annette
  Palliative Medicine (2006), 118
  Seven deaths in Darwin: case studies (1998), 115, 119
Stroke, 80–81, 144, 152
Stuart, Paul
  Pope John Paul II and the Redemptive Power of Suffering (2005), 194
St. Vincent's Hospital, Melbourne
  Tonti-Filippini, 76, 111, 137, 172
Substituted consent, 134, 136–138
Substitute Judgement, 8, 37–38, 121–138, 200

Suffering
  capacity to suffer, 72
  cause for despair, 162
  cause growth, 159
  Christ, 169
  Christian understanding of, 162
  deepening our understanding, 160
  desire to live, 115
  empathy, 72
  existential, 65, 178–180
  finds dignity, 162
  happiness, 161–162
  incapacity, 164
  Jesus, 162
  joy, 162
  loneliness, 178
  loss of function, 164
  mystery of, 161
  occasion of hope, 162
  peace, 162
  perplexing, 162, 164
  personal growth, 72
  philosophers, 159
  problem of, 159
  reason, 162
  redemption, 194
  secular understanding of, 162
  solitary, 168
  source of wisdom, 160
  suppresses capacity to reason, 164
  the human condition, 159
Suicidal, 30, 78, 86, 92, 94, 101, 136, 145
Suicidal project, 87, 89
Suicide
  abetting suicide, 30, 94, 123, 131, 136
  aiding suicide, 31, 94, 123, 131, 136
  facilitate, 94
  physical-assisted, 21
  prevent, 30–31, 86–87, 94–95, 131, 136
  psychological evaluation, 114
  reasonable force to prevent, 94
Suicide by omission
  person's refusal, 87

Support of others
  dying, 118
  serious illness, 118
Supreme Court of Western Australia, 85
Survival in Cancer Patients Undergoing in-hospital Cardiopulmonary Resuscitation: a Meta-Analysis, 77
Swallow food
  tube feeding, 80
Symptoms, 17, 19, 41, 45, 56, 66, 86, 88–90, 112, 149, 179, 198

Taboo, 45
Taylor, Charles T.
  The Ethics of Authenticity (1992), 127
Technology, 10, 27, 48, 52, 58, 65–67, 118, 159, 181
Teleology, 28
Ten, Chin Liew Mill
  On Liberty (2001), 33
Tenderness, 20
Teresa Benedicta, St. (Bl. Edith Stein), 191
Terminal Illness
  mercy-killing, 107
  palliative care, 106
Termination of pregnancy, 53
The American Journal of Bioethics, 145
The Lancet (1998), 115, 119
Theologians, 74, 164, 176, 193
Theological Studies in Marriage and Family, 111
Theological Virtues
  believers, 182
  charity, 185
  Christians, 22
  faith, 21, 24, 178
  hope, 21, 24, 178
  love, 21, 24, 179
  non-believers, 182
Therapy
  chemotherapy, 75, 184
  electro-convulsive therapy, 155
  psychotherapy, 155
  radiotherapy, 75

Index   227

Thomas Aquinas, St.
 a posteriori, 166
 Aristotelian, 166
 form and matter, 166
Tissue, 10, 52, 58, 62, 123, 164, 192
Tolerance, 19, 140, 188
Tonti-Filippini, Claire, 172
Tonti-Filippini, John, 9
Tonti-Filippini, Justin, 9, 163
Tonti-Filippini, Lucianne, 9
Tonti-Filippini, Nicholas
 Angina, 76, 116
 Autobiographical, 173–174
 Director of Bioethics, 111
 haemodialysis, 116, 199
 health insurer, 112
 John Paul II Institute, 10, 111
 mass, 167
 Monash University, 111, 176–177
 my illnesses, 9, 110, 197
 Nancy (Filippini, Contessa), 172
 National Health and Medical
  Research Council, 40, 46, 52, 58, 100,
  111, 123
 philosopher, 5
 University of Melbourne, 111, 125
Torres Strait Islander, 20, 46
Torture, 10
Tosolini, Dr Andrew, 189
Total Parenteral Nutrition, 80
Tradition
 manualistic tradition, 26
Tragedy, 6, 71, 172
Transgender surgery, 53
Treatment
 burdensome treatment, 74, 78,
  97, 199
 coercive treatment, 155
 dummy treatment, 155
 emergency treatment, 30, 87, 93
 fatal treatment, 96, 100
 futile treatment, 7
 life prolonging treatment, 86, 109
 medical treatment, 122–124

 psychiatric treatments, 155
 refusing treatment, 101
Tribunal, 36, 91–92, 95, 132, 141, 152
Trinitarian Anthropology, 159,
  165–167, 171
Trinitarian Mystery, 166
Trinity
 communio personarum, 166
 communion of persons, 170, 173
 trinitarian anthropology, 159, 165
 trinitarian love, 165
Trust, 9, 24, 28, 39, 47, 50, 98, 102, 105,
  138–140, 146–147, 195, 197
Trusteeship, 34
Truth, 2–3, 5–6
Truth-Telling
 deception, 155
Tube Feeding
 act of love, 83
 discomfort of, 83
 economic rationalism, 84
 spoon-feeding, 84
 surgical procedure, 80, 83
Tube Feeding and Persistent Vegetative
  State Patients: Ordinary or
  Extraordinary Means?, 74

Understanding
 lack of, 46
Unethical, 8, 50, 52–54, 88, 103, 105
Unique, 11, 51, 106, 166, 173
United Nations
 euthanasia, 119
 Human Rights Committee, 119
United Nations Convention against
  Illicit Traffic in Narcotic Drugs and
  Psychotropic Substances, 132
United Nations Convention against
  Transnational Organised Crime, 132
United Nations International Covenant on
  Civil and Political Rights, 54, 62, 99,
  119, 124, 129
United Nations International Covenant
  on Economic, Social and Cultural

Rights, 132
United Nations Protocol to prevent suppress, and punish trafficking in persons, especially women and children, 132
United States, 29, 63, 106
Unity, 23, 99, 166, 168, 170, 172–173, 187, 194
University of Melbourne, 111, 125
Unresponsive state
  conscious, 82, 99, 111, 176, 193
US State of Oregon
  Oregon Phase Two, 68
Utilitarianism Ethics, 67
Utilitiarian, 12, 67, 178
Utilitiarianism
  for and against, 67

Valium, 43, 77
Values
  personal, 18
Van Delden JJ
  Lancet 1991, 110
Van Der Maas PJ
  Lancet 1991, 110
Vatican
  catechism, 72
  catholic, 72
  Christian, 171
  Church, 171
  Gaudium et Spes, 24, 161
  John Paul II, 24
Vegetable, 82
Vegetative State
  unresponsive state, 176
Victoria Community Protection Act (1988), 157
Victoria Medical Treatment Act (1988), 94, 122–123, 131, 146
Victorian Disability Act (2006), 122
Victorian Guardianship and Administration Act (1985)
Victorian Guardianship and Administration Act (1986), 134

Victorian Law Reform Commission
  decision-making capacity, 124, 127
  impairments, 128
Victorian Medical Treatment Act (1998), 94, 122–123, 131, 146
Victorian Mental Health Act (1986), 122, 133
Victorian Scrutiny of Acts and Regulations Committee, 59, 61
Victorian Supreme Court, 137
Vocation
  celibate, 168
  communion, 127
  marriage, 171
  professional, 50
  spouse, 168
  to love god, 168

Waclaw
  Auschwitz, 1940–1945, 88
Wadell, Charles
  MJA 165 (540), 110
Wallace SK
  Resuscitation (2006), 77
Walsh, Mary, 9, 15, 17, 22–24, 76, 165, 167, 174, 182, 184, 186, 192–197
Water
  hydration, 81, 84
  refusal of, 84–85
Webb FJ
  Resuscitation (2006), 77
Weiss, Matthew D., 145
Well-being, 65–66, 68, 91, 127, 134, 139
White, Thomas Joseph
  Jesus' Cry on the Cross, 163
Will
  advanced directive, 92
  legal, 86
  living will, 92
Williams, Bernard
  Utilitarian: for and against (1973), 67
Wilson GR
  Resuscitation (2006), 77

Wolf, Susan M
  Feminism and Bioethics (1996), 114
Woods v. Lowns and Procopis, 42
Works of God, 161, 191
World Health Organisation
  International Classifications of
    Diseases (ICD-10), 152
  well-being, 65
World Medical Association,
    102–103

www.ingramcontent.com/pod-product-compliance
Lightning Source LLC
Chambersburg PA
CBHW070349240426
43671CB00013BA/2446